# Cuddling A

## PICTURE BO

CW01468164

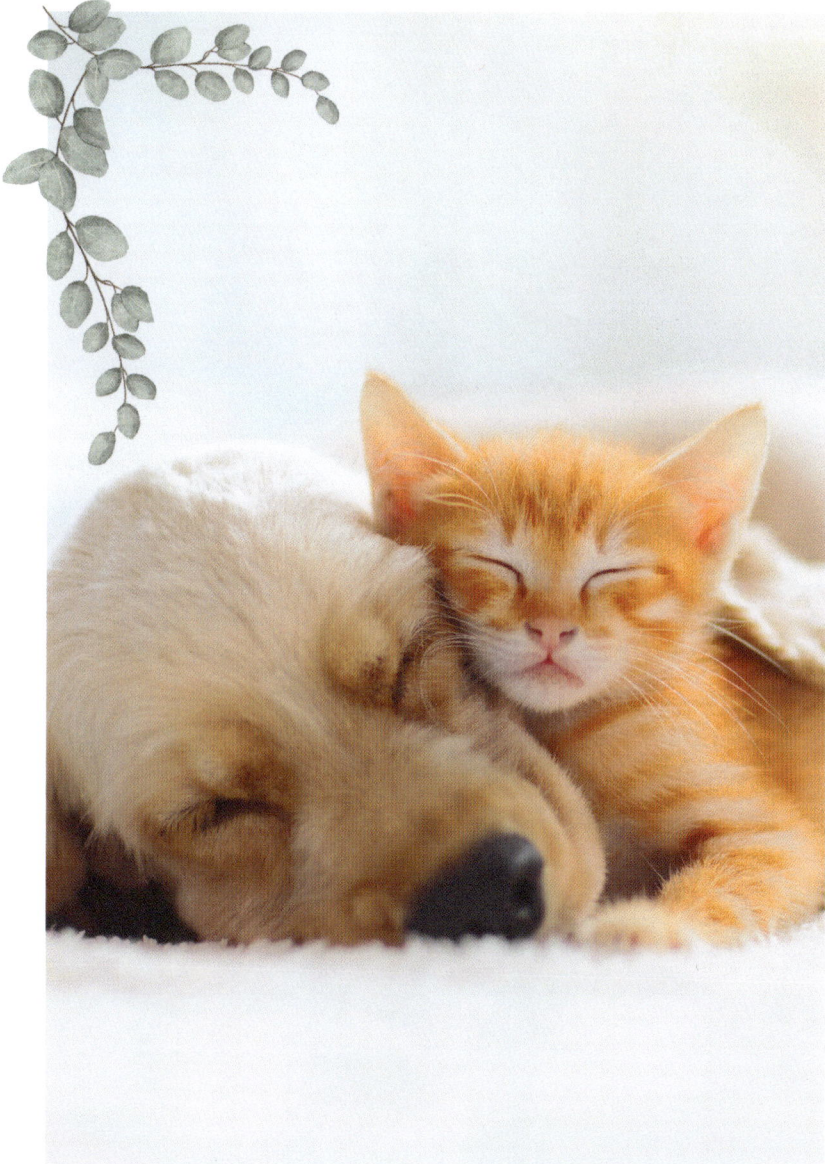

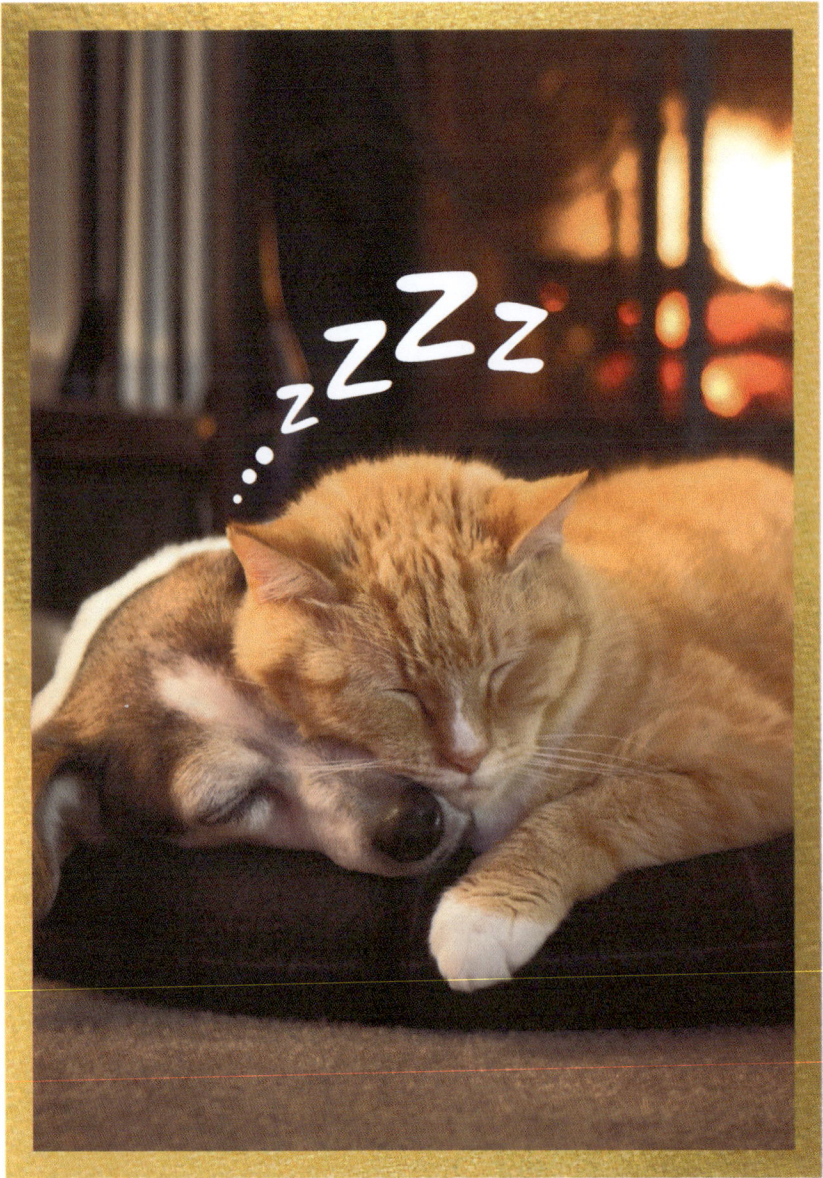

*zzZz*

So nice to have a friend like you

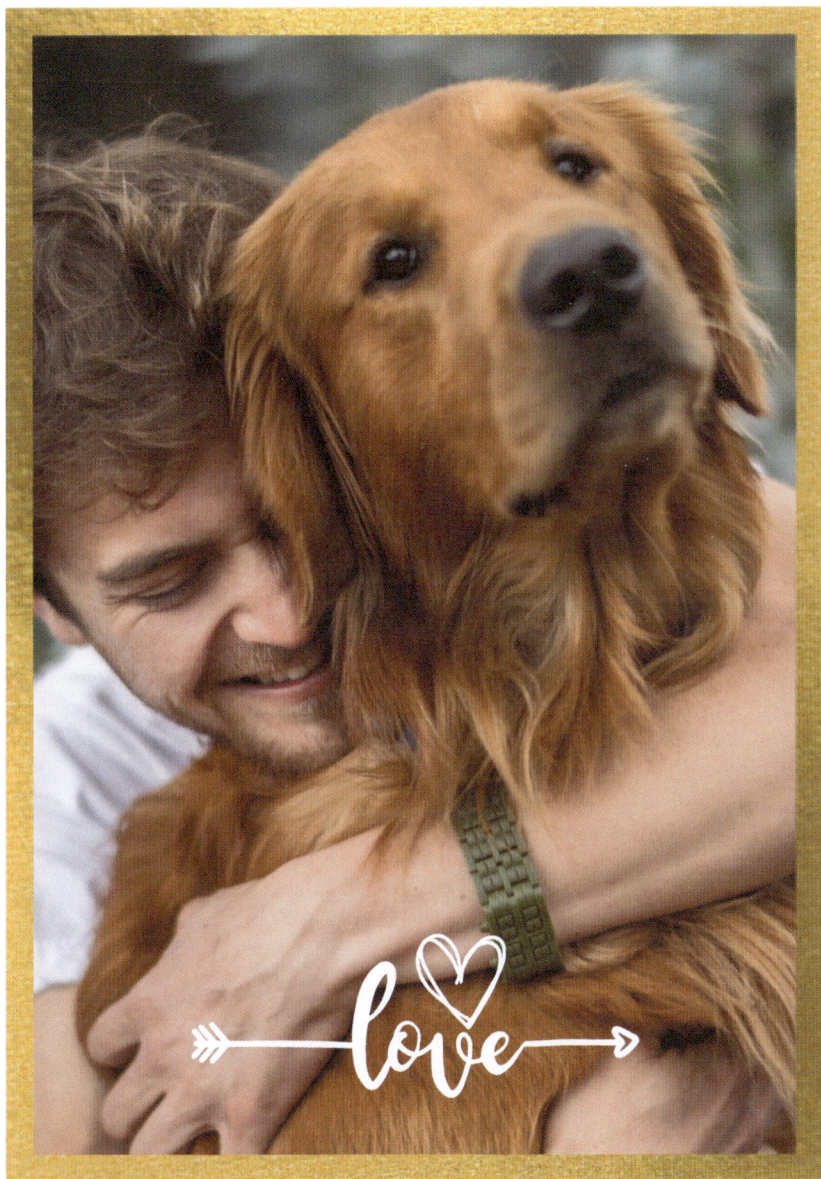

love

Bro. I love you.

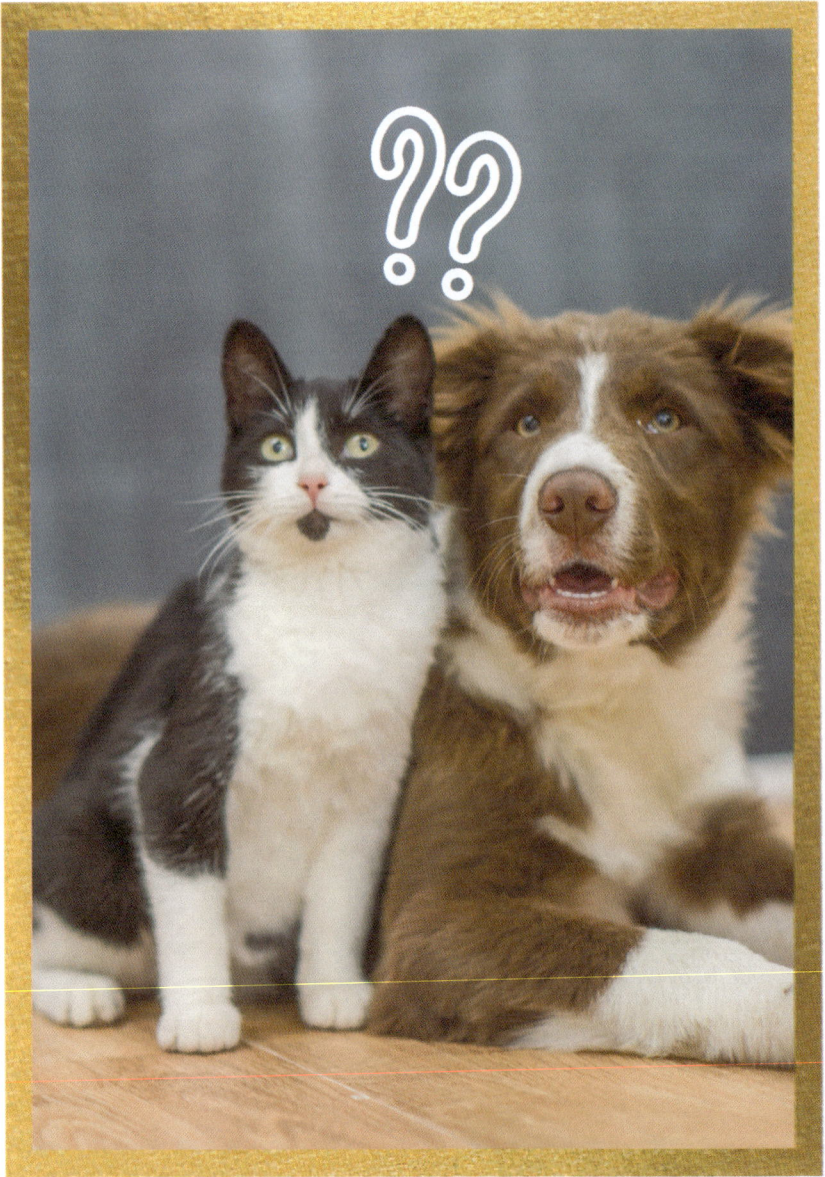

What are you saying?

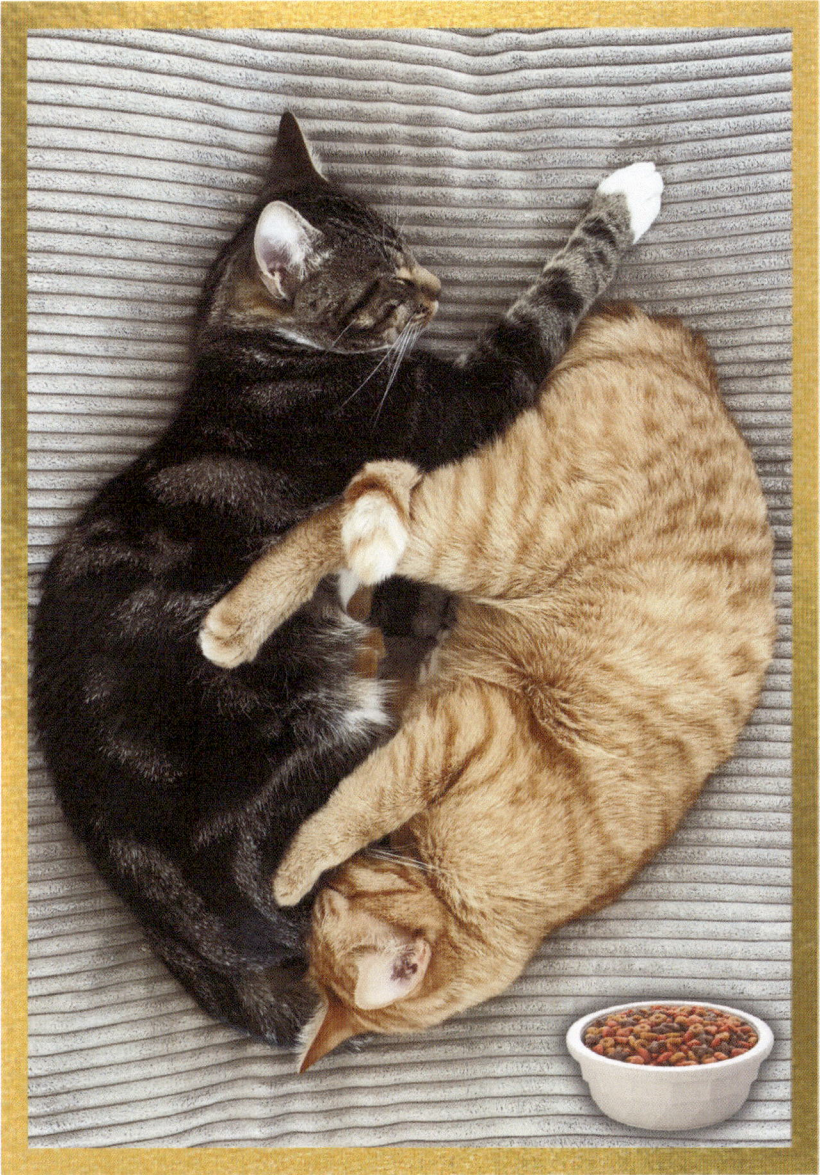

We smell each other's butt

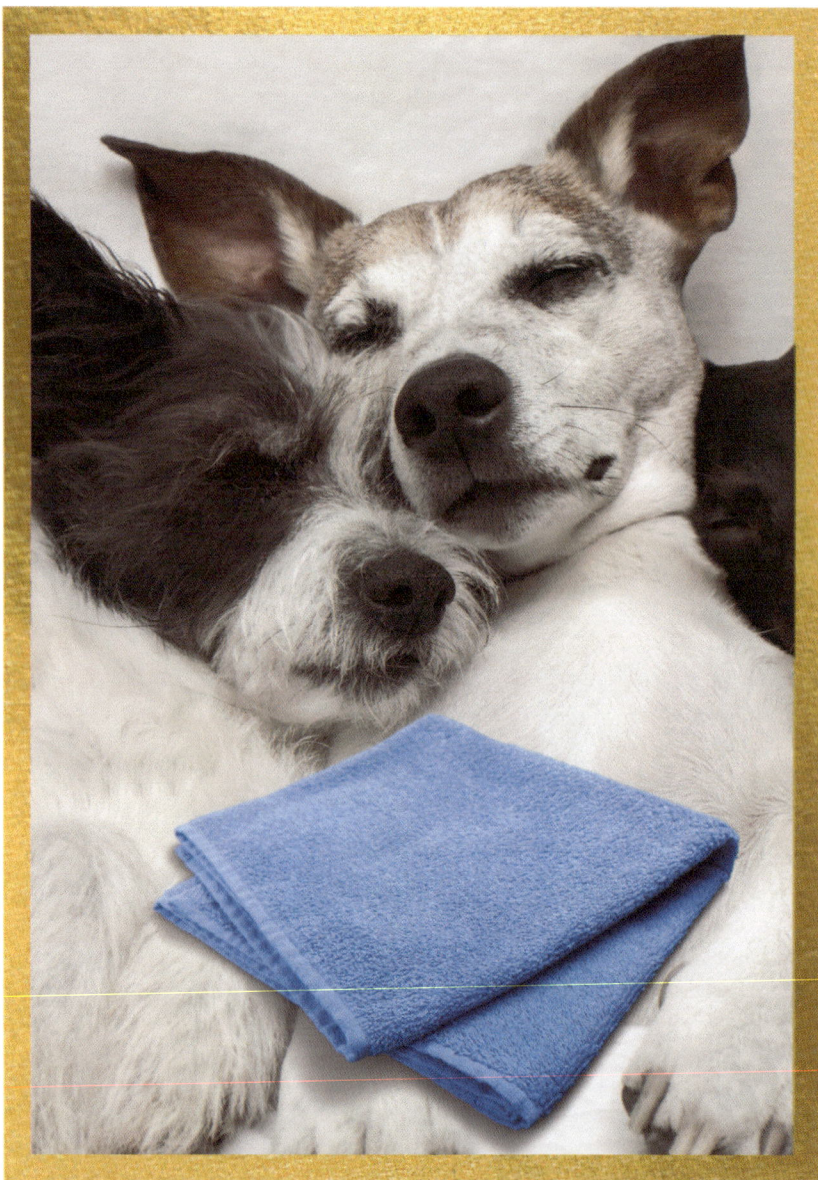

Sorry folks. Simply too tired... Zzz ...

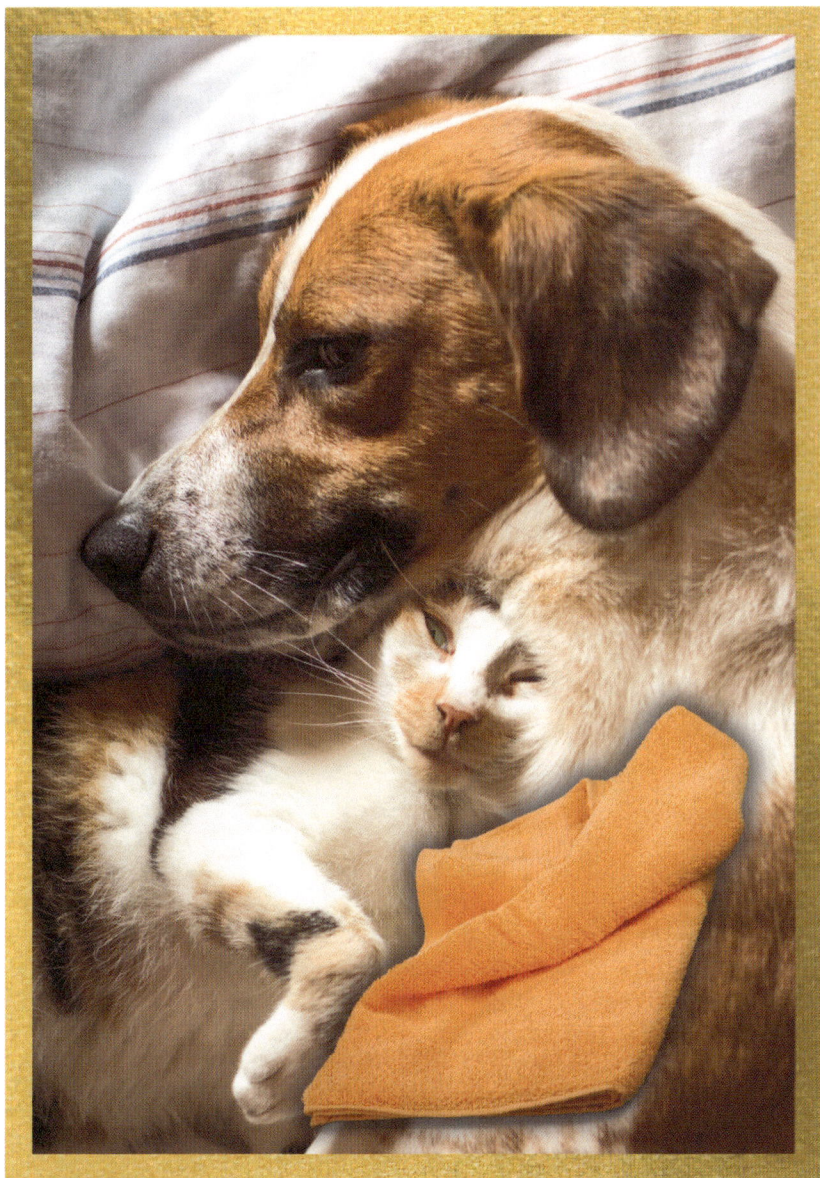

No worry. I'll protect you.

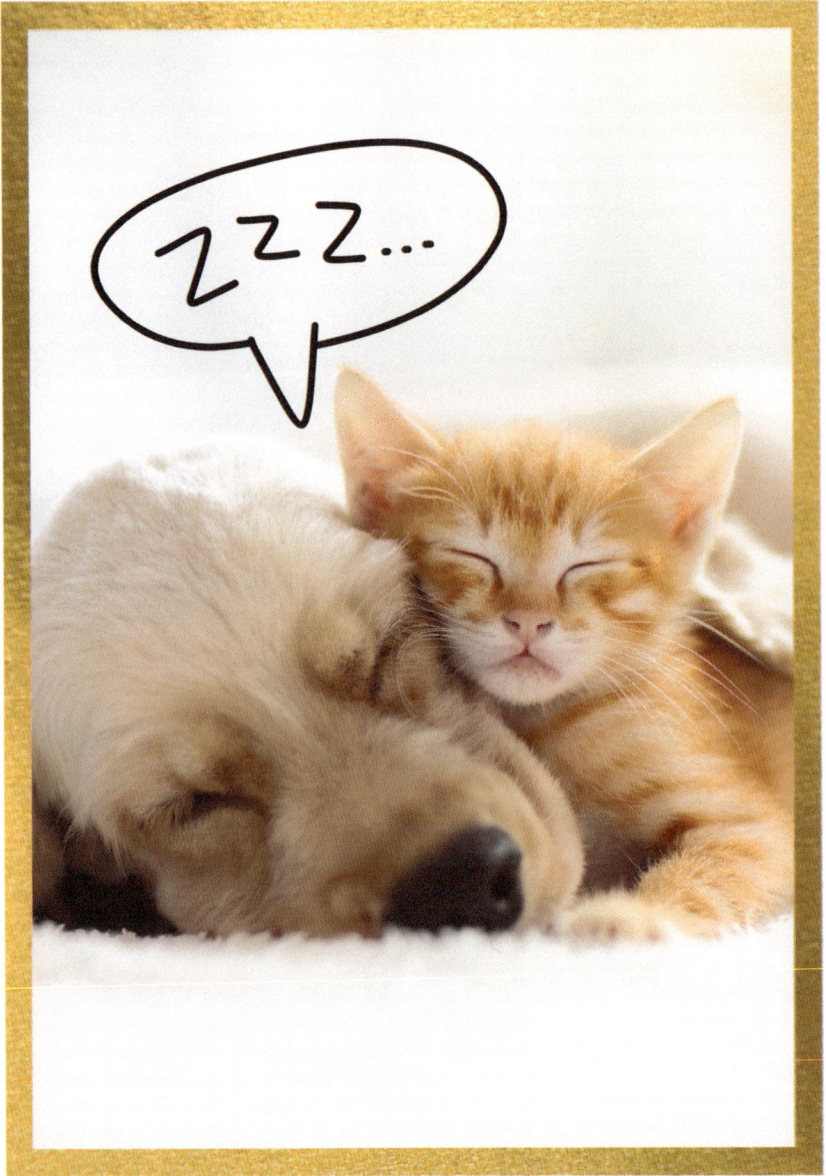

Shh ... We are having a nice nap

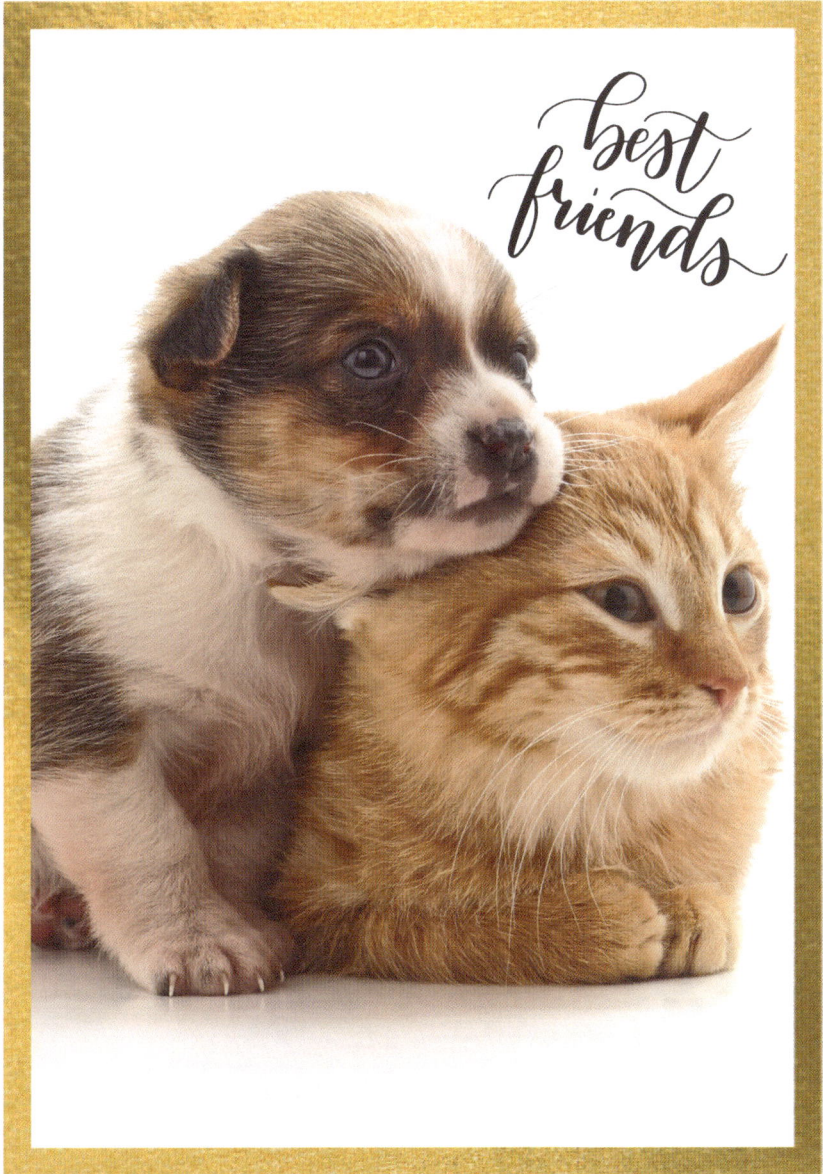

best
friends

Aren't we compatible?

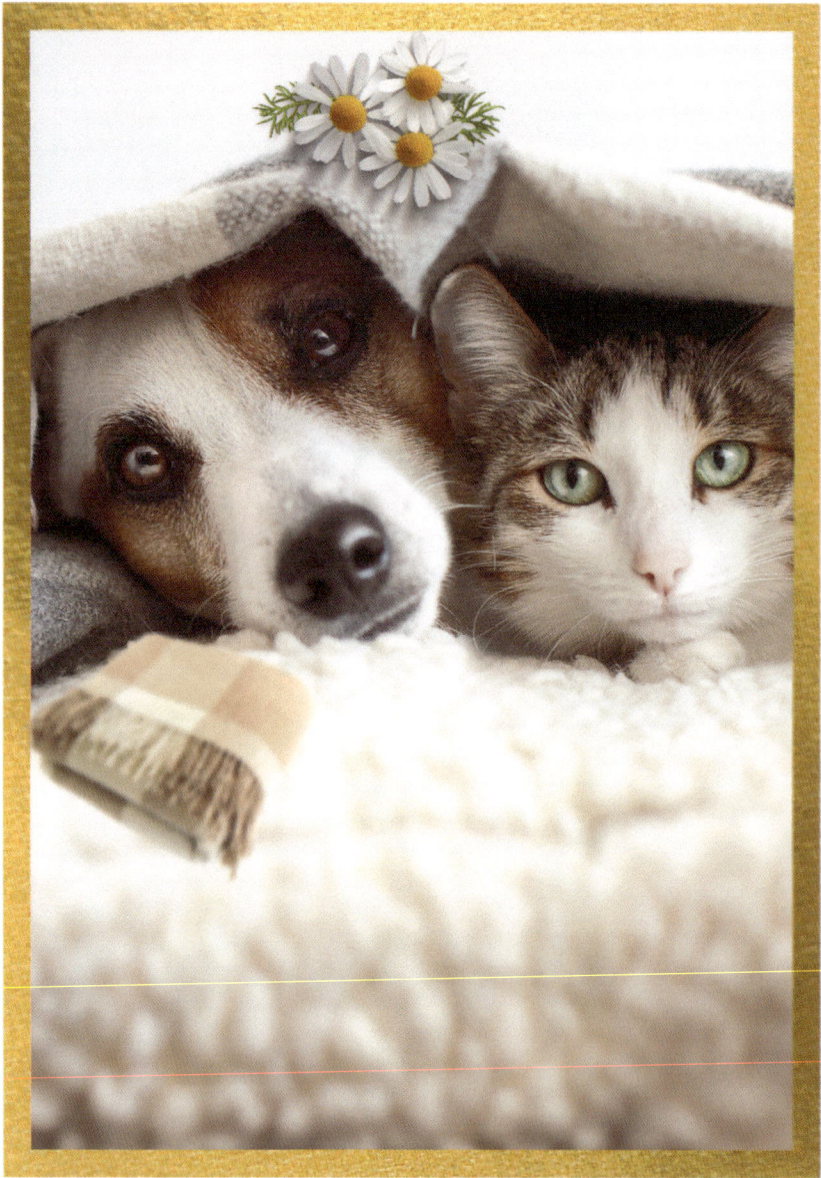

Under one blanket

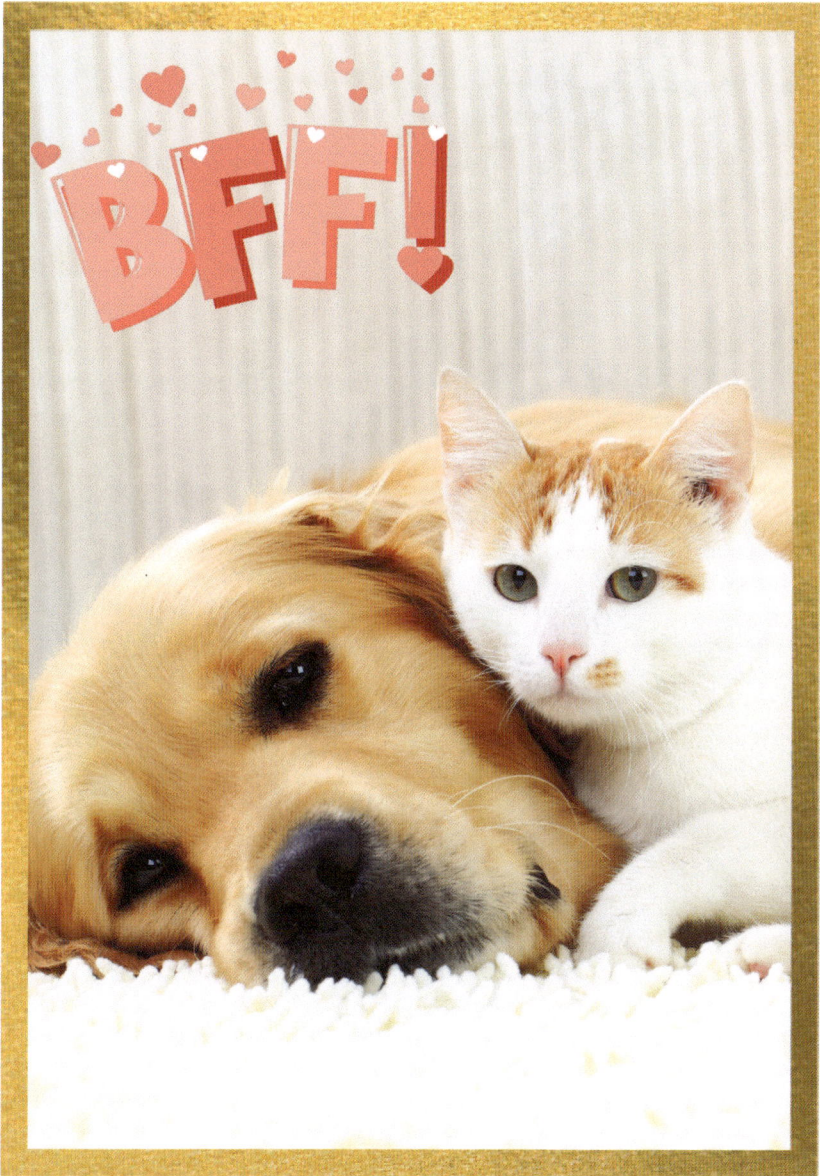

**BFF!**

We are best friends

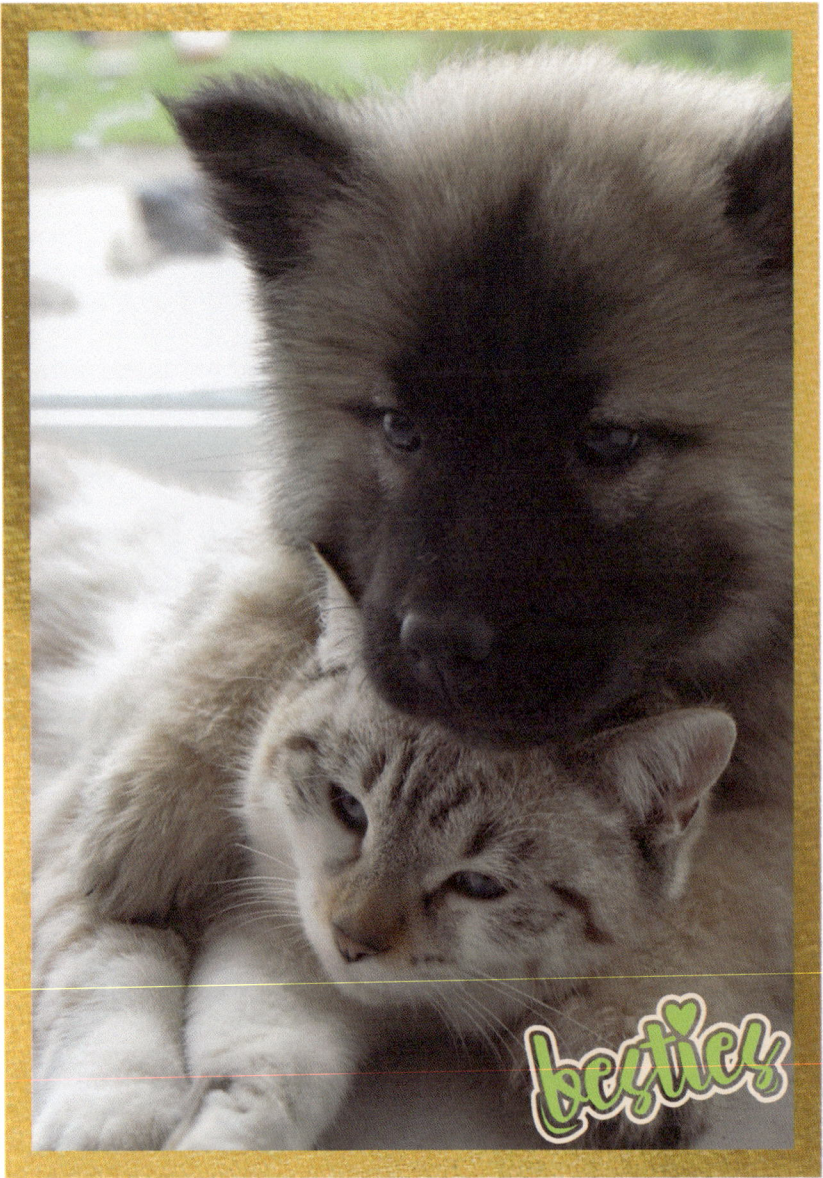

besties

We are friends forever

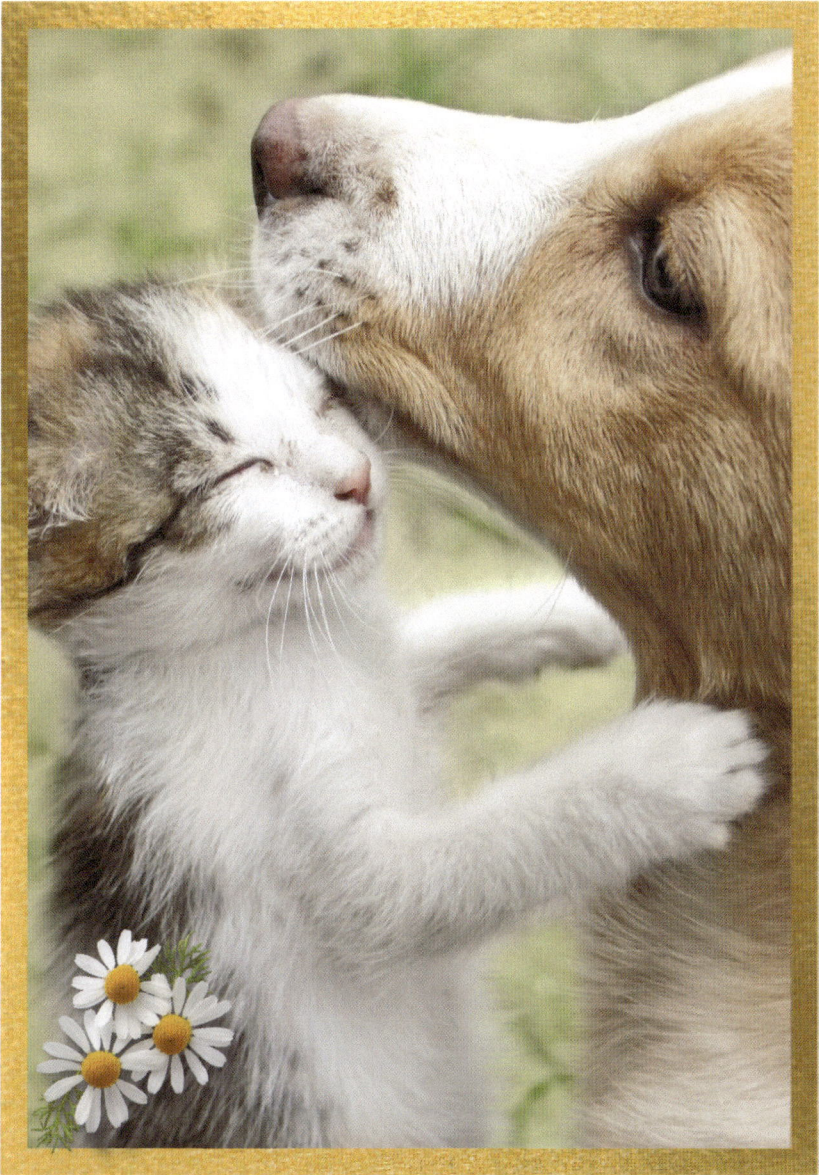

Come on. Let's have a hug

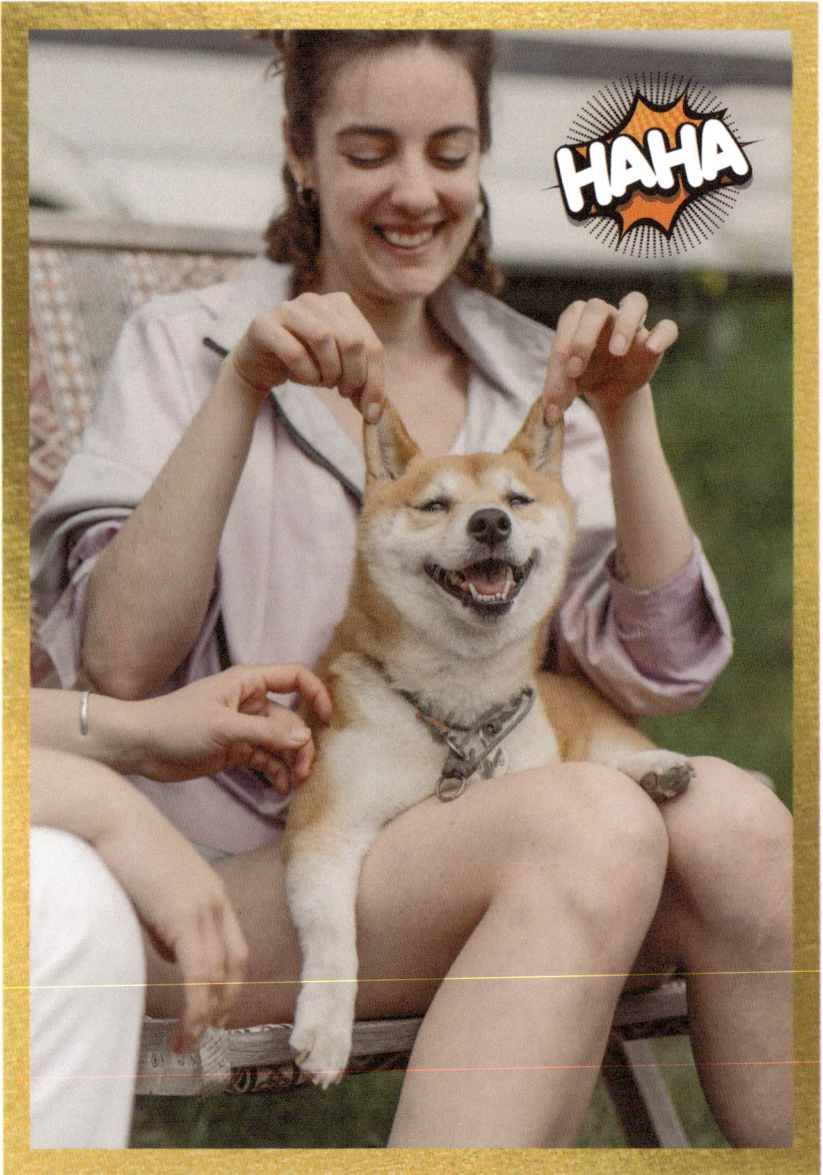

I have nice ears right?

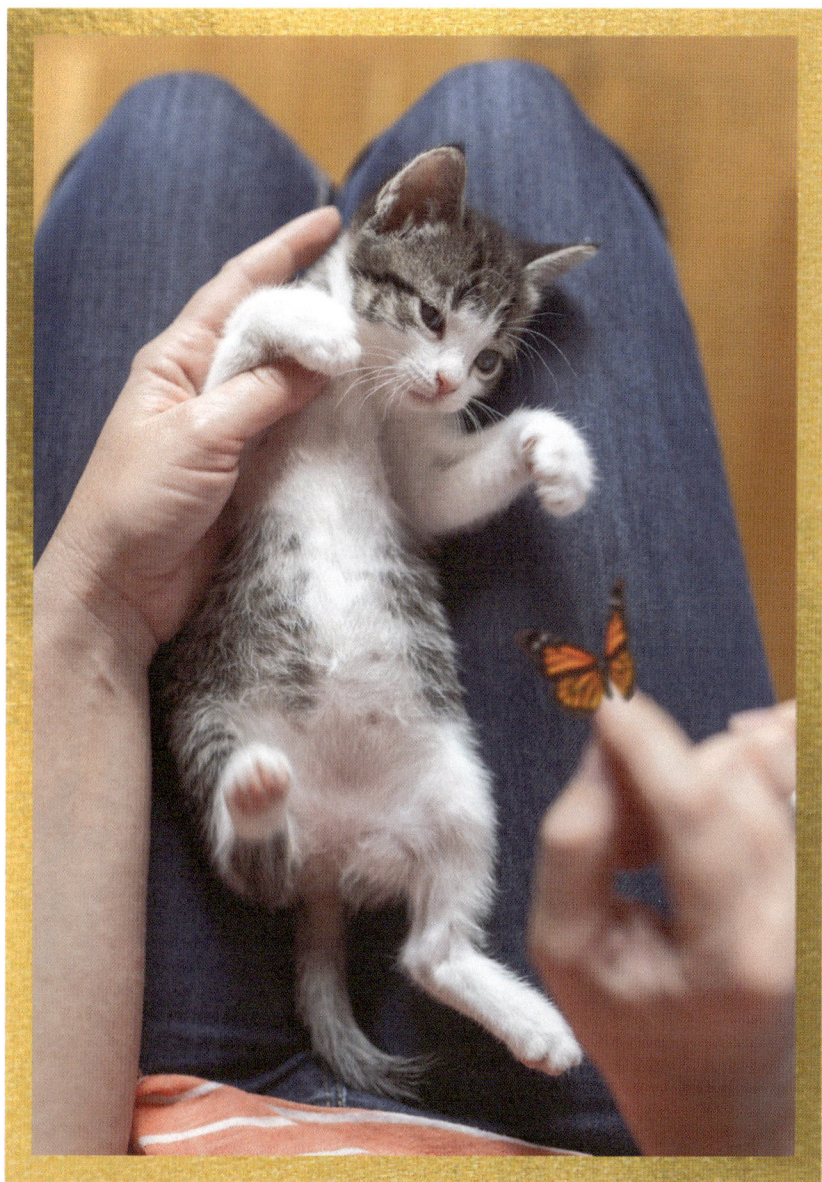

Don't you tickle me!

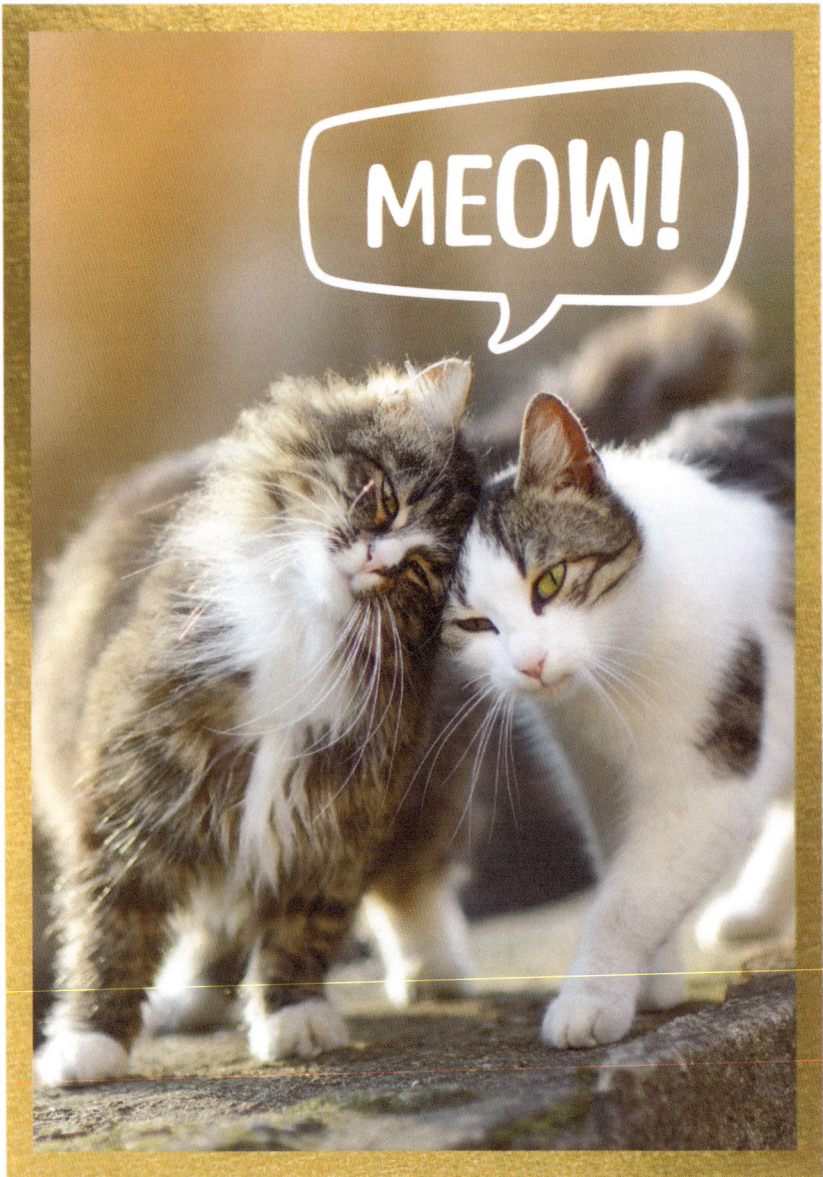

That's how we show friendship

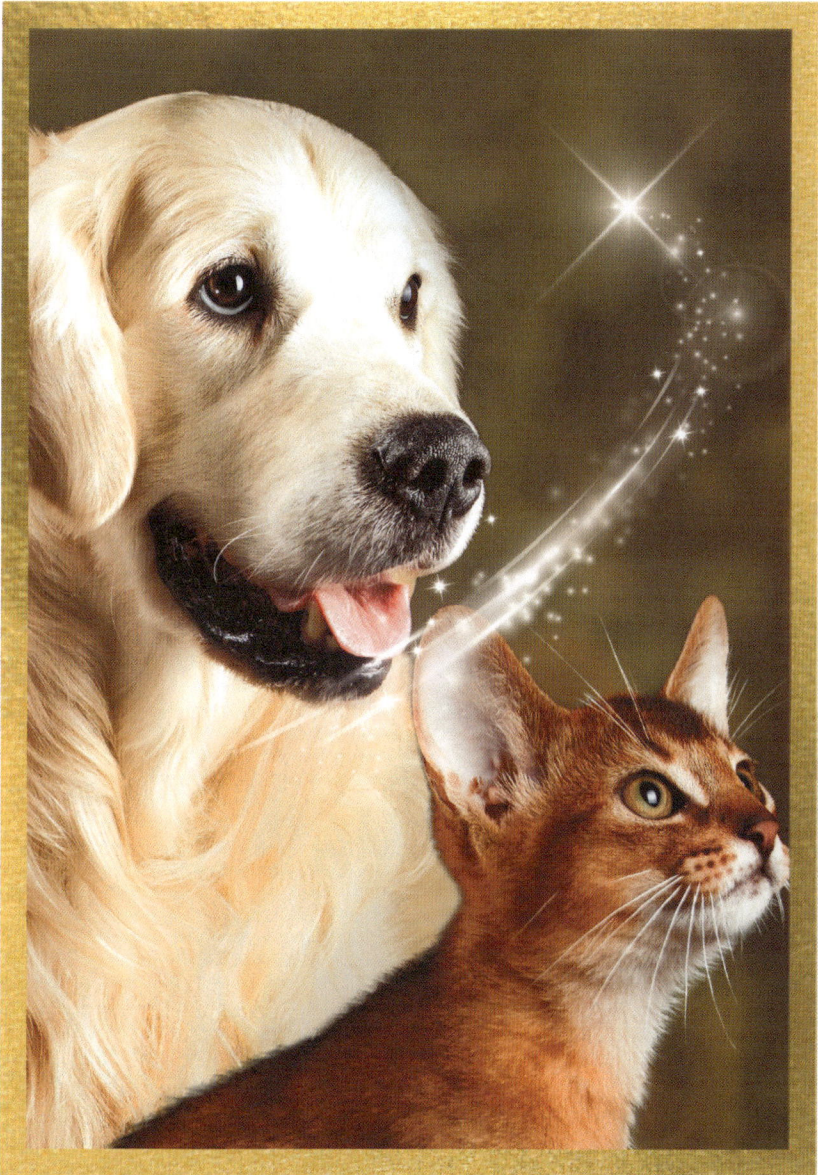

We will have a future!

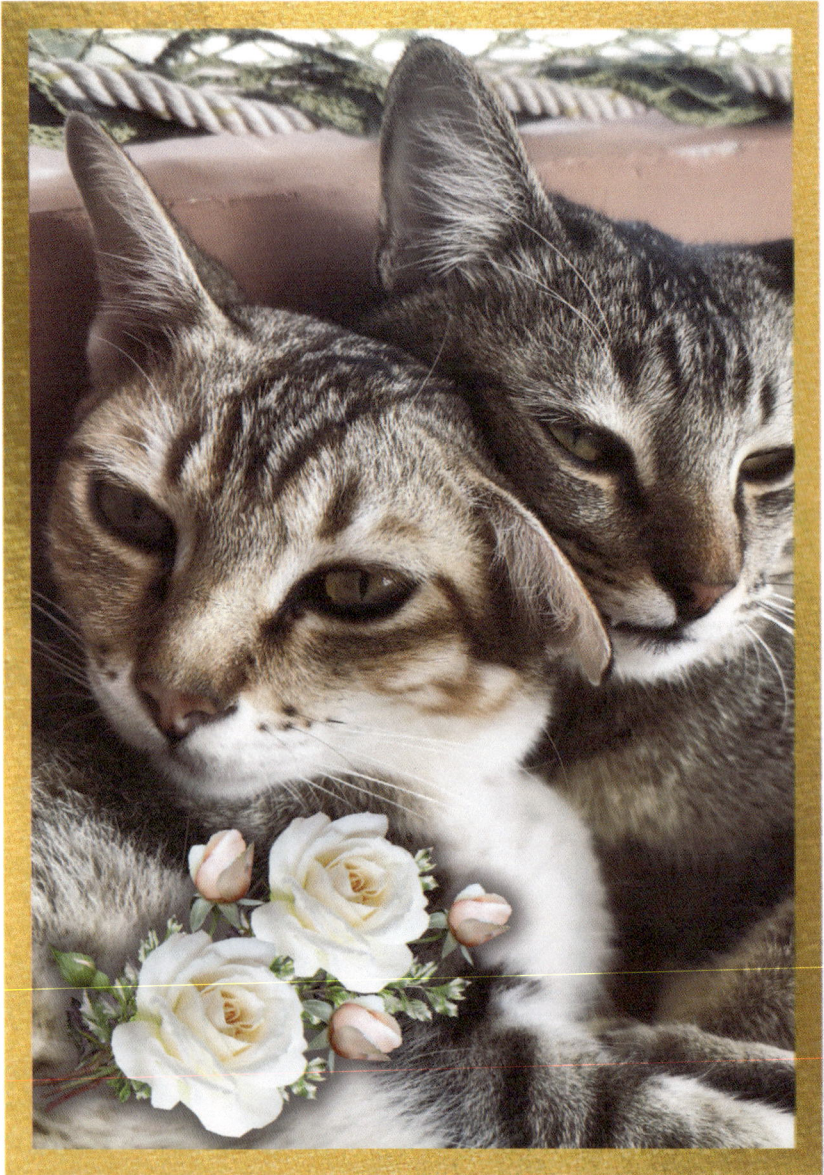

Who is calling? We want to sleep

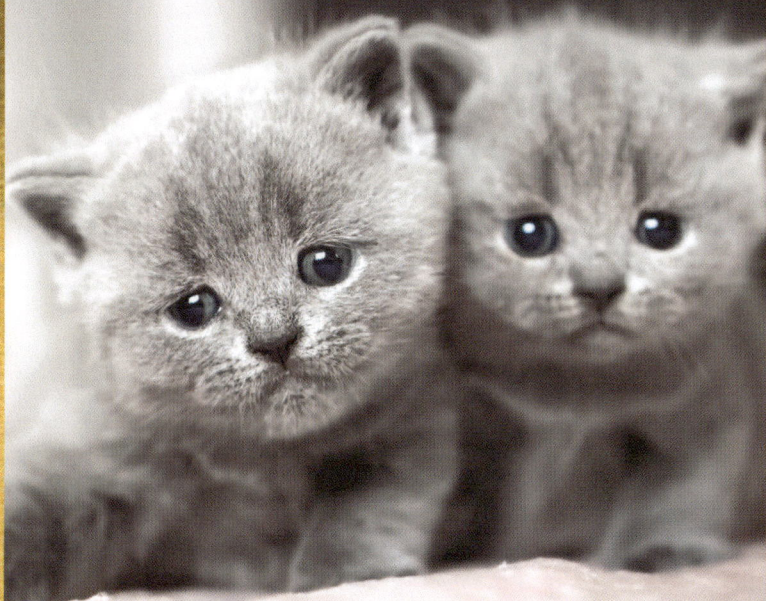

miss you

When is mom coming back?

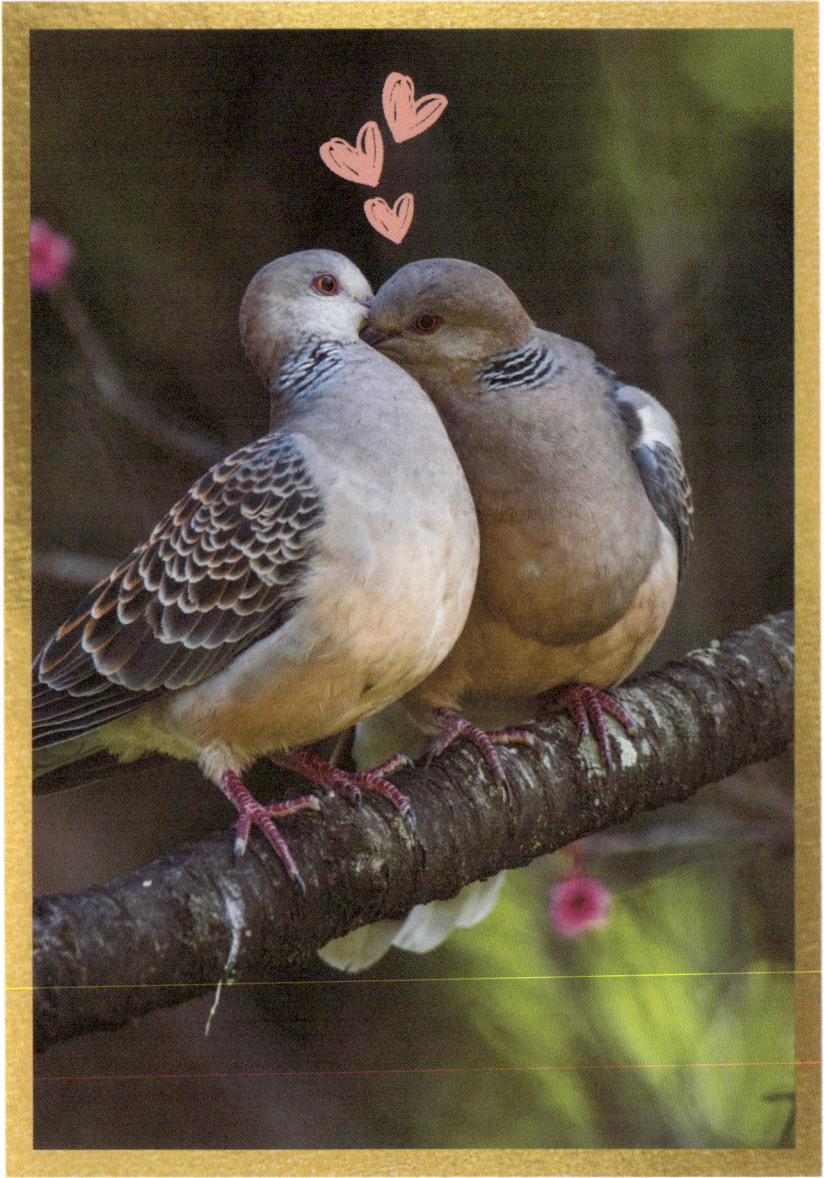

You smell good

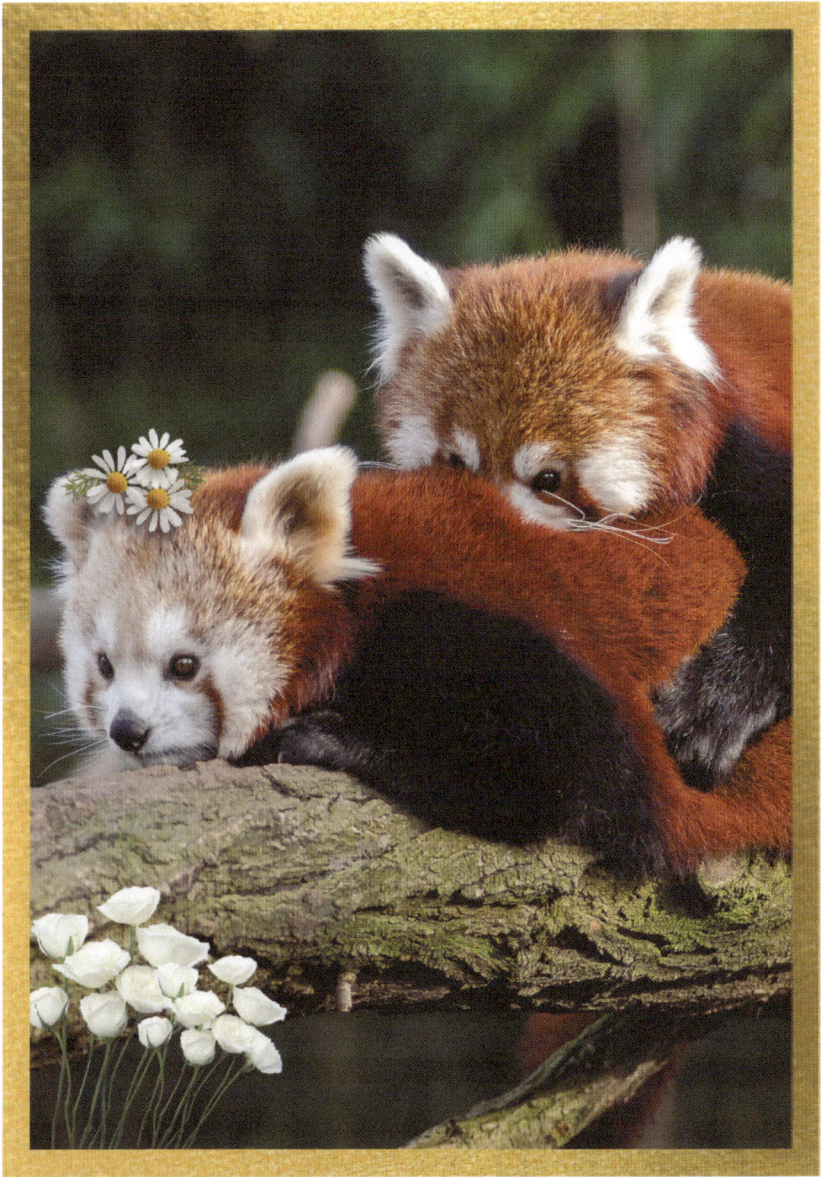

Smelling you out!

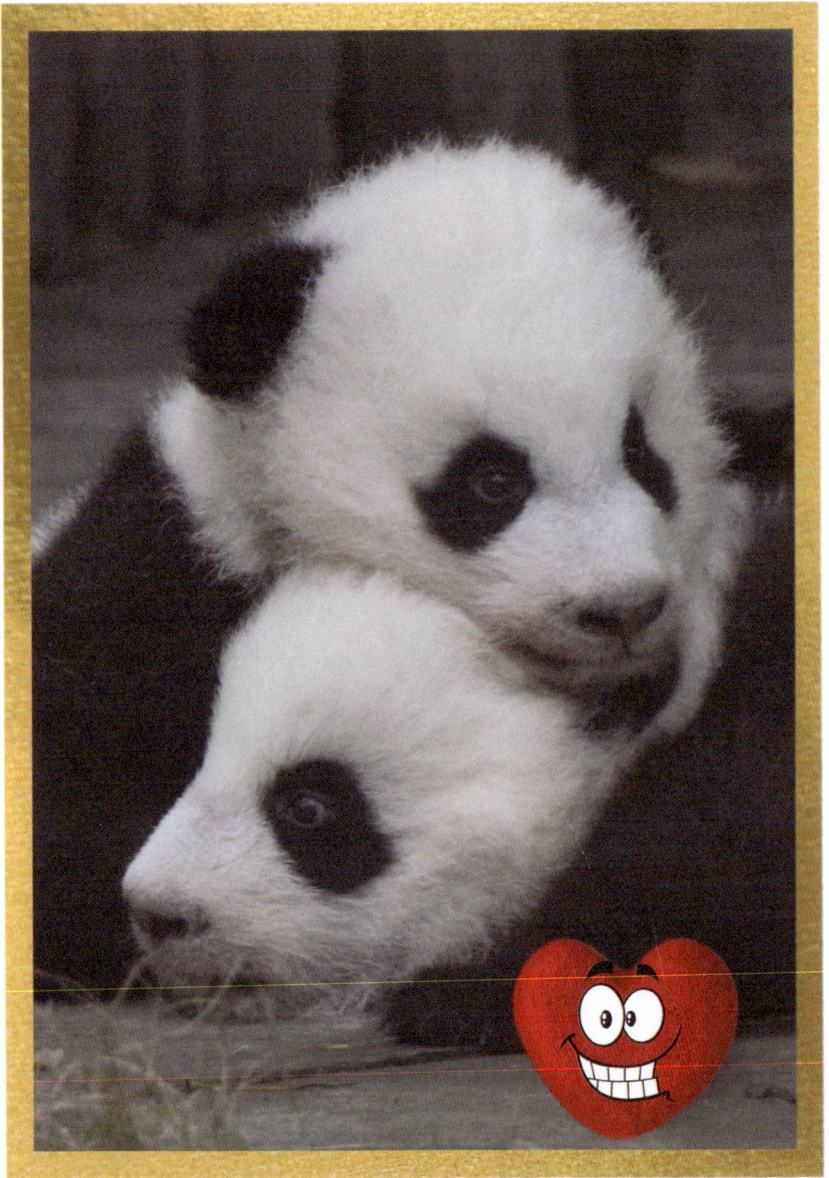

Can you be my pillow?

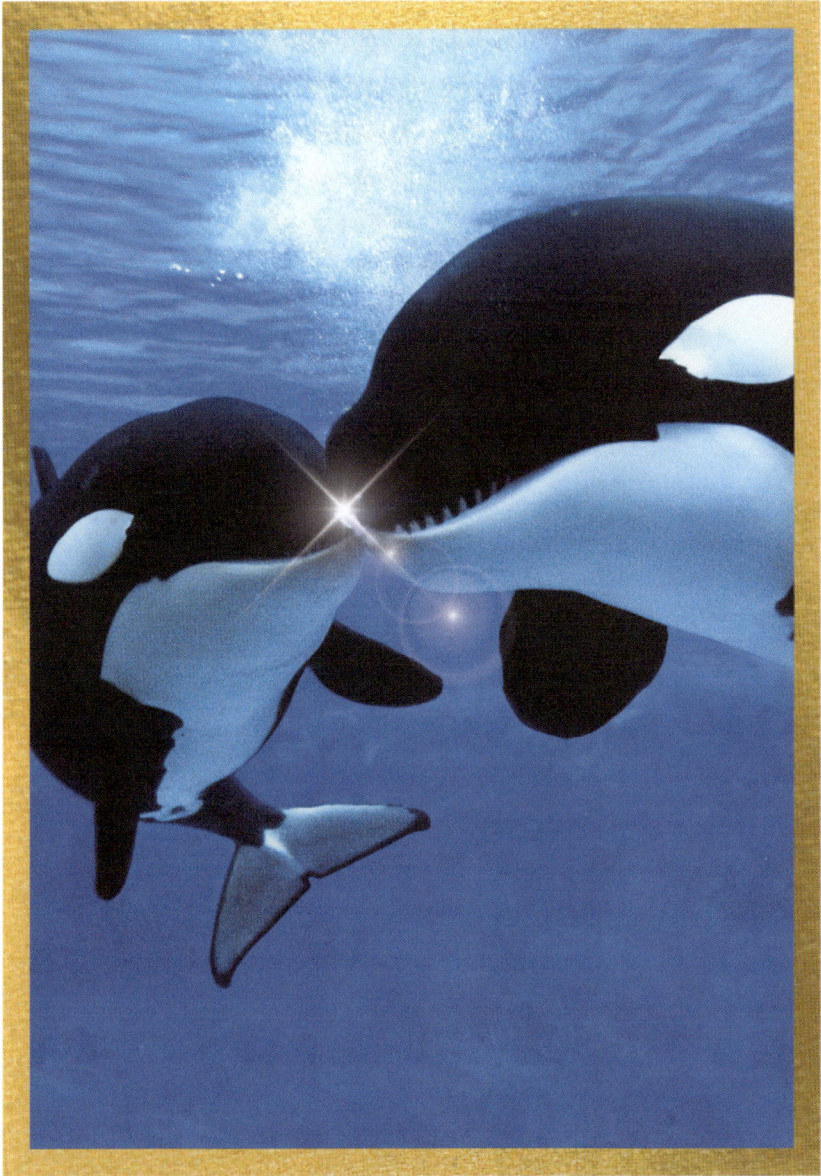

Love in ocean

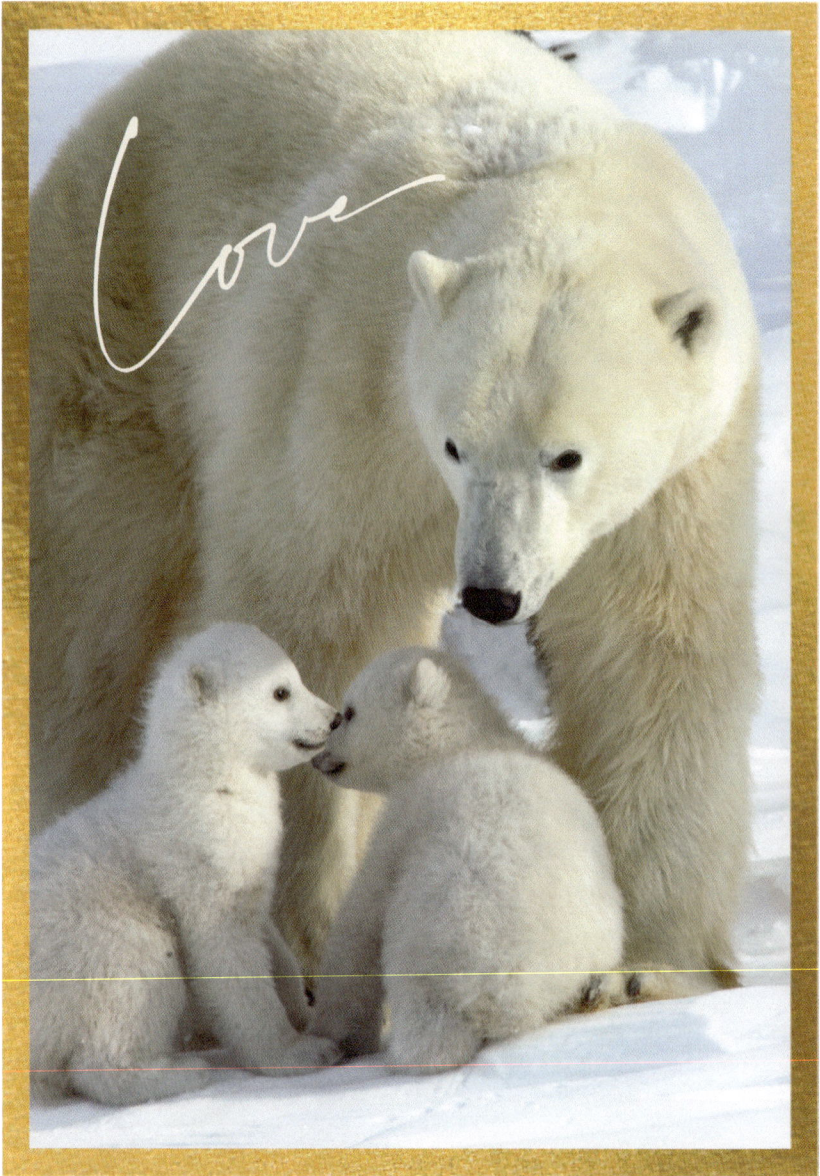

*Love*

We are a family

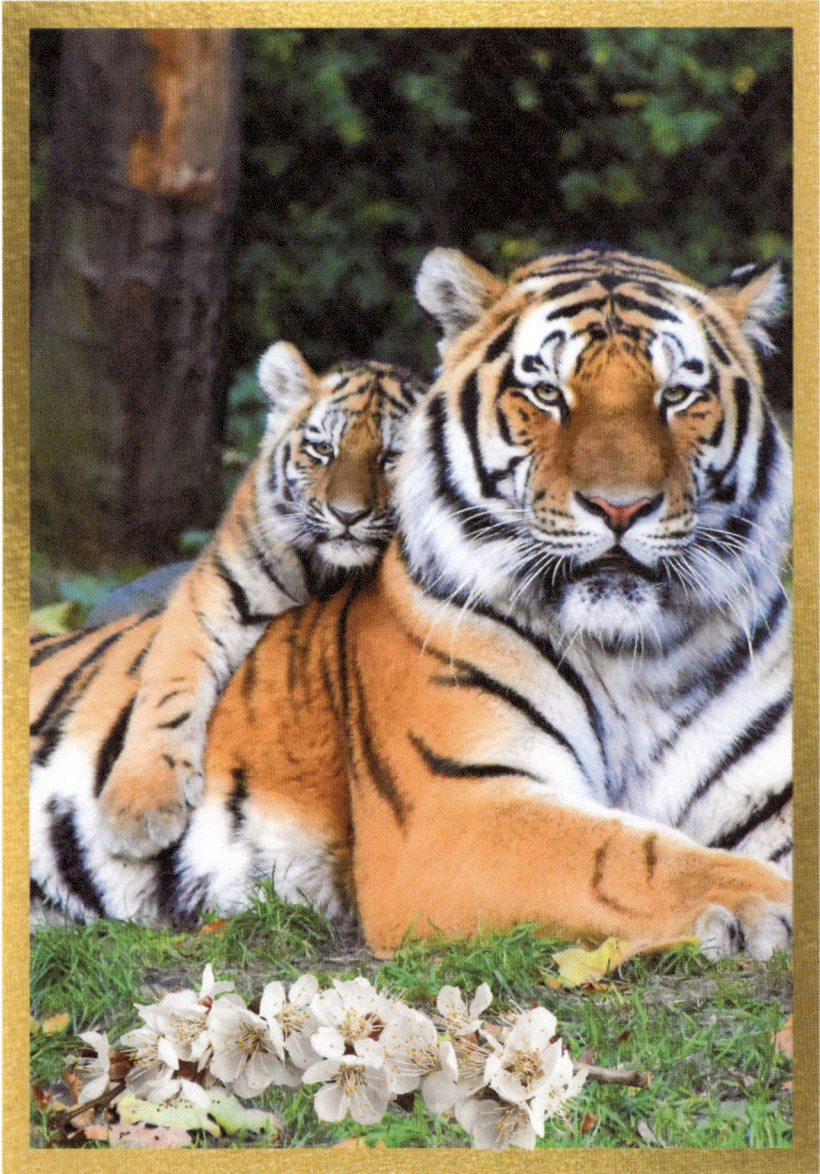

Mom is the best!

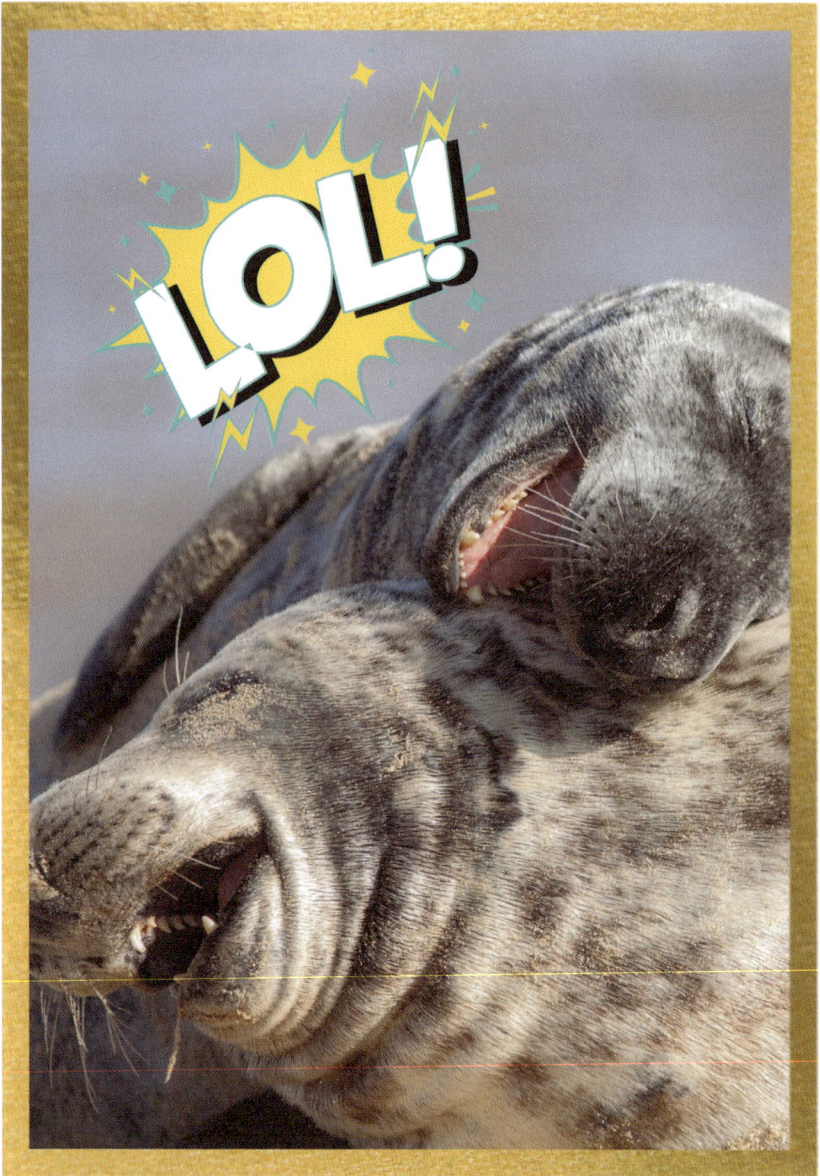

What a hiliarious joke!

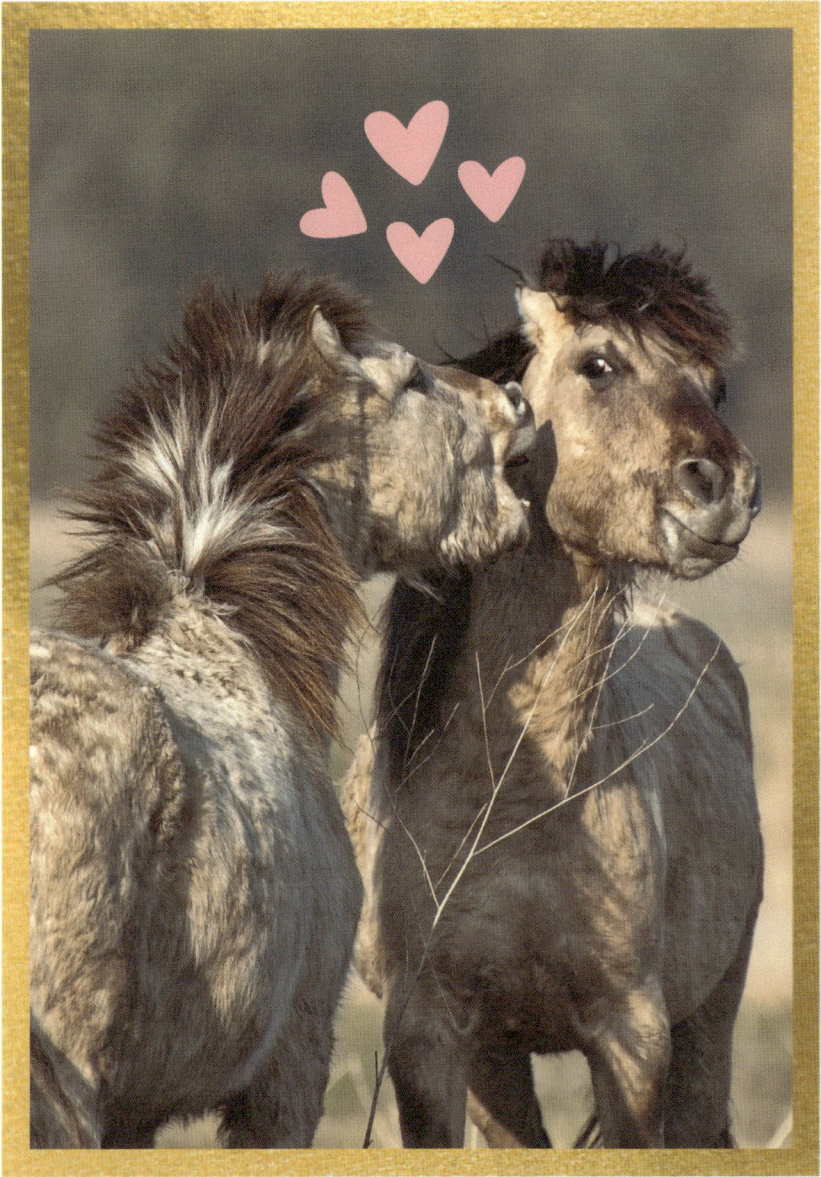

Don't be shy sweetie

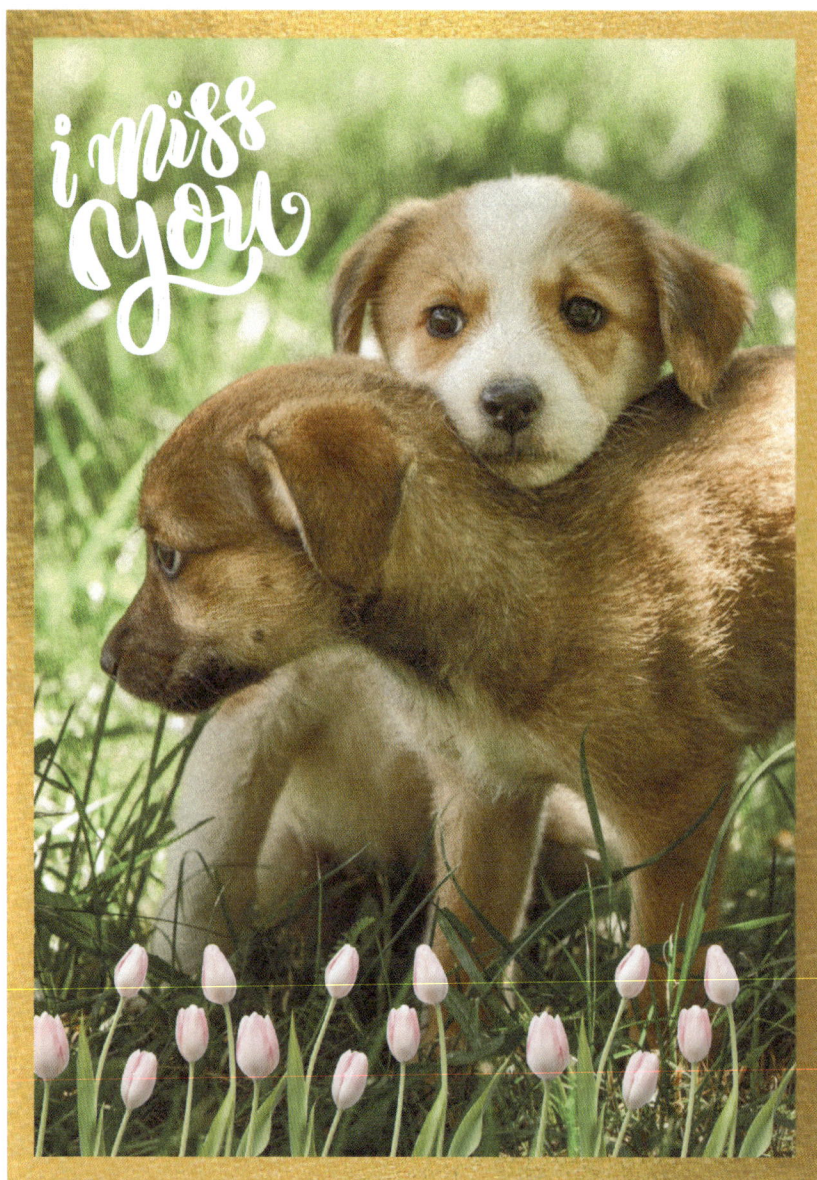

i miss you

Where is mom?

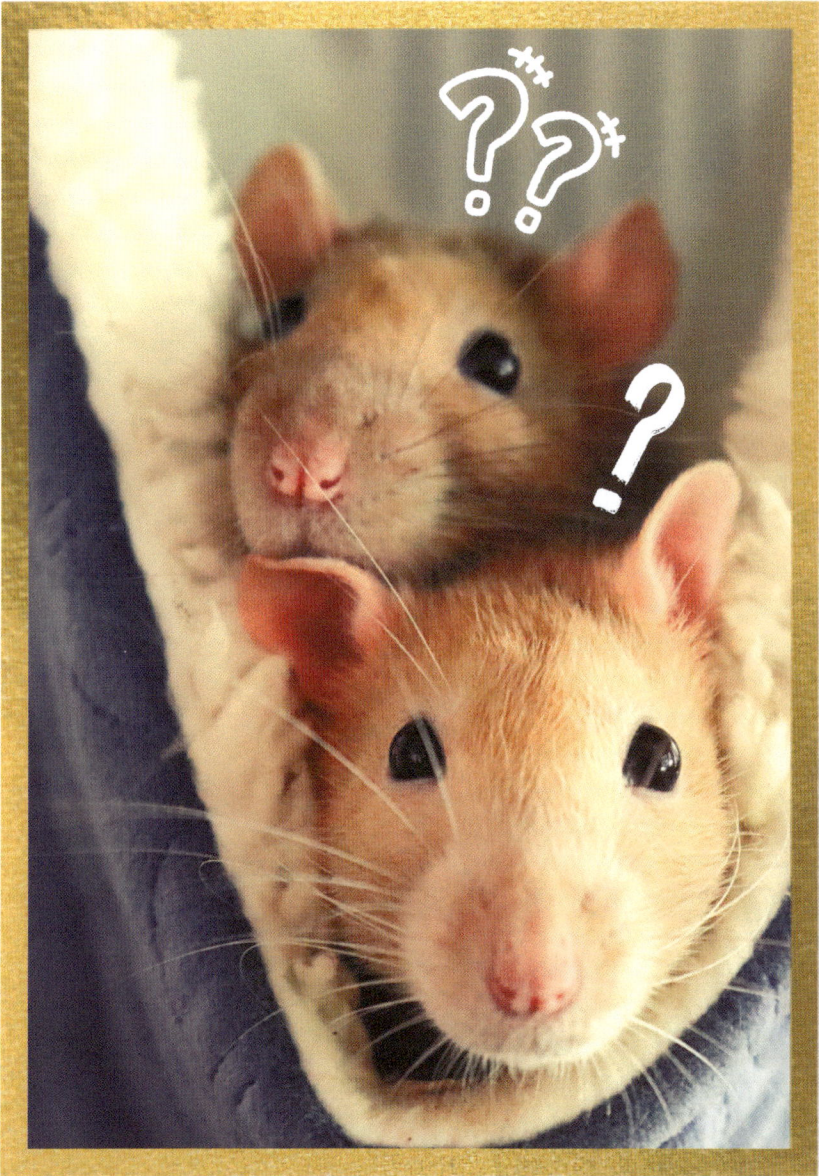

Anyone out there?

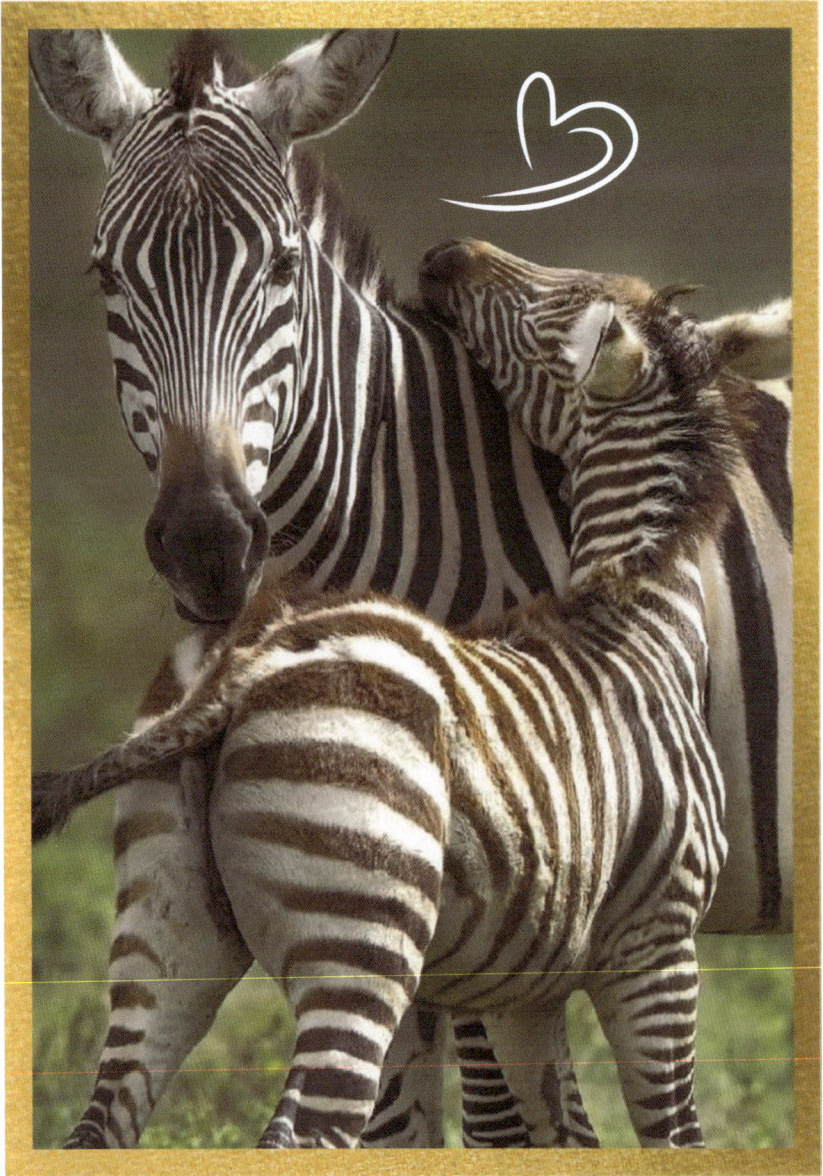

Mom I miss you!

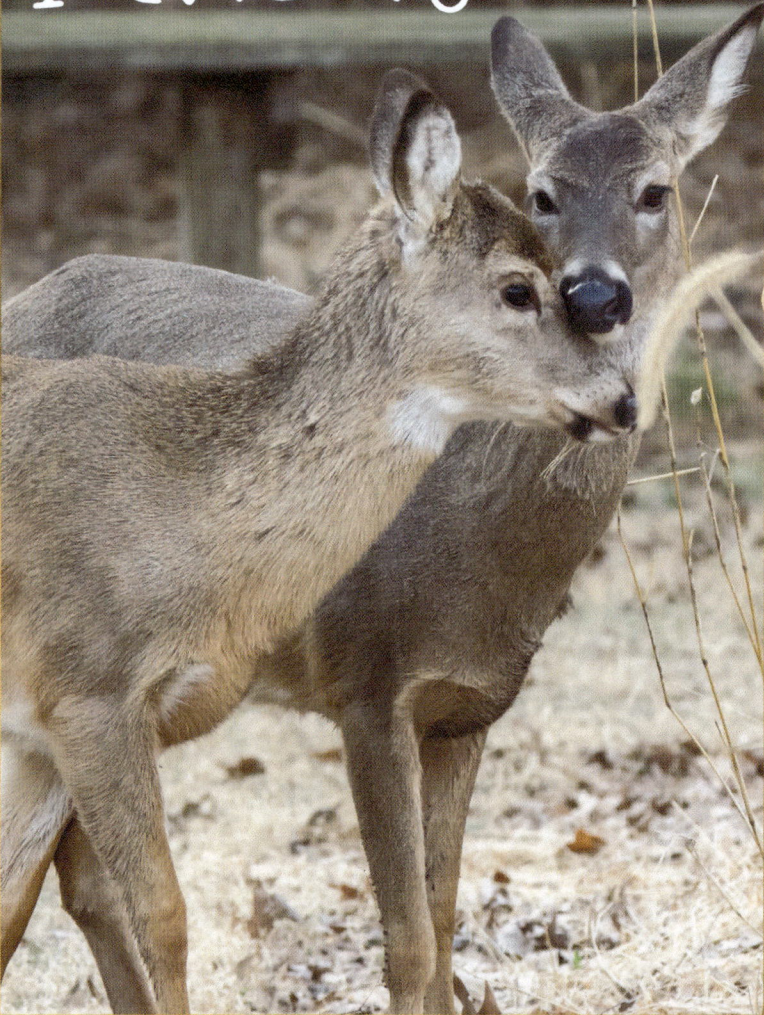

I LOVE YOU

Where have you been?
I miss you a lot!

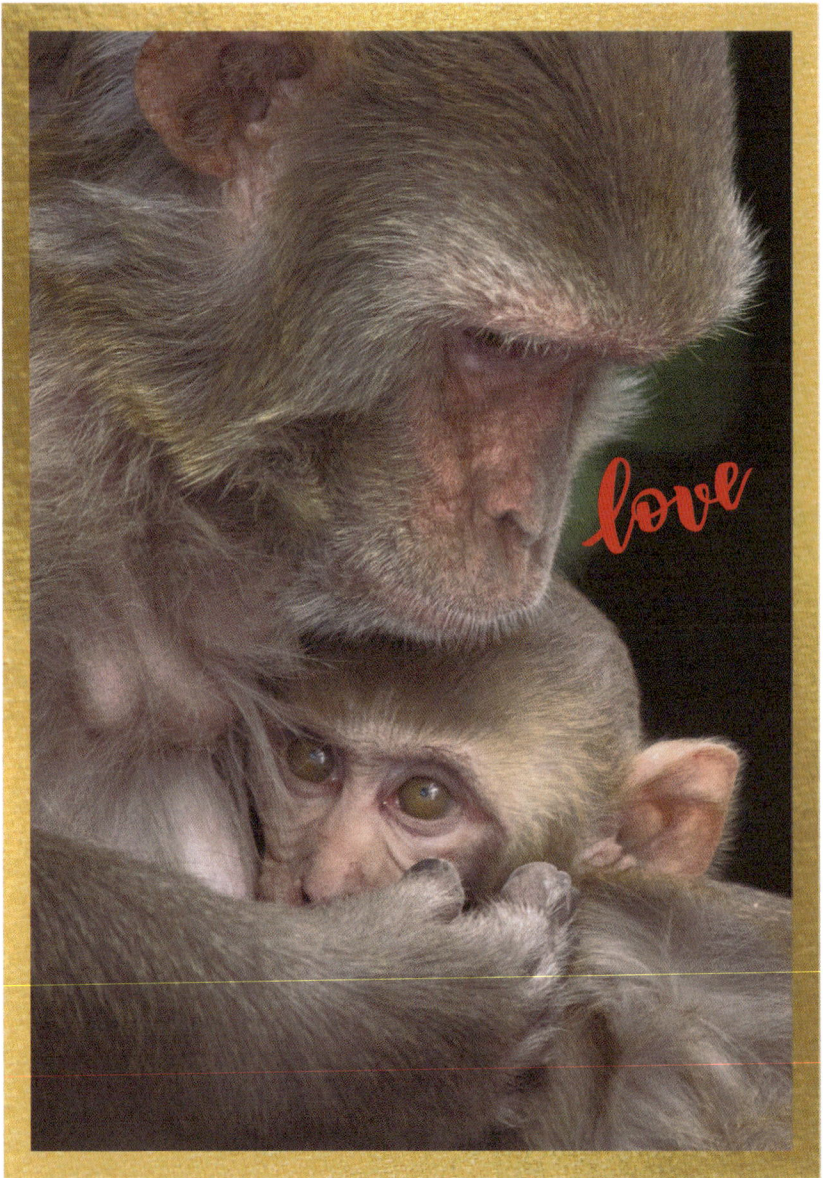

love

Good girl. Mom loves you.

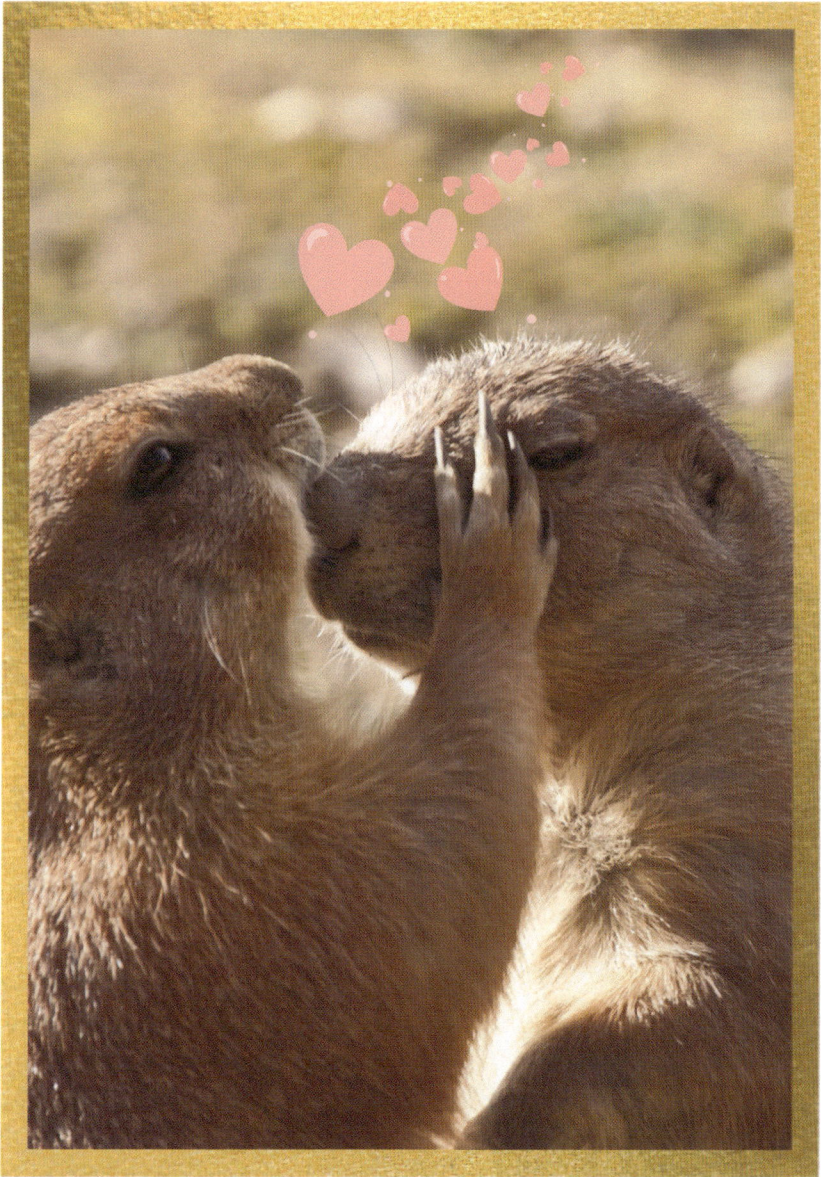

Let me clean your eyes for you

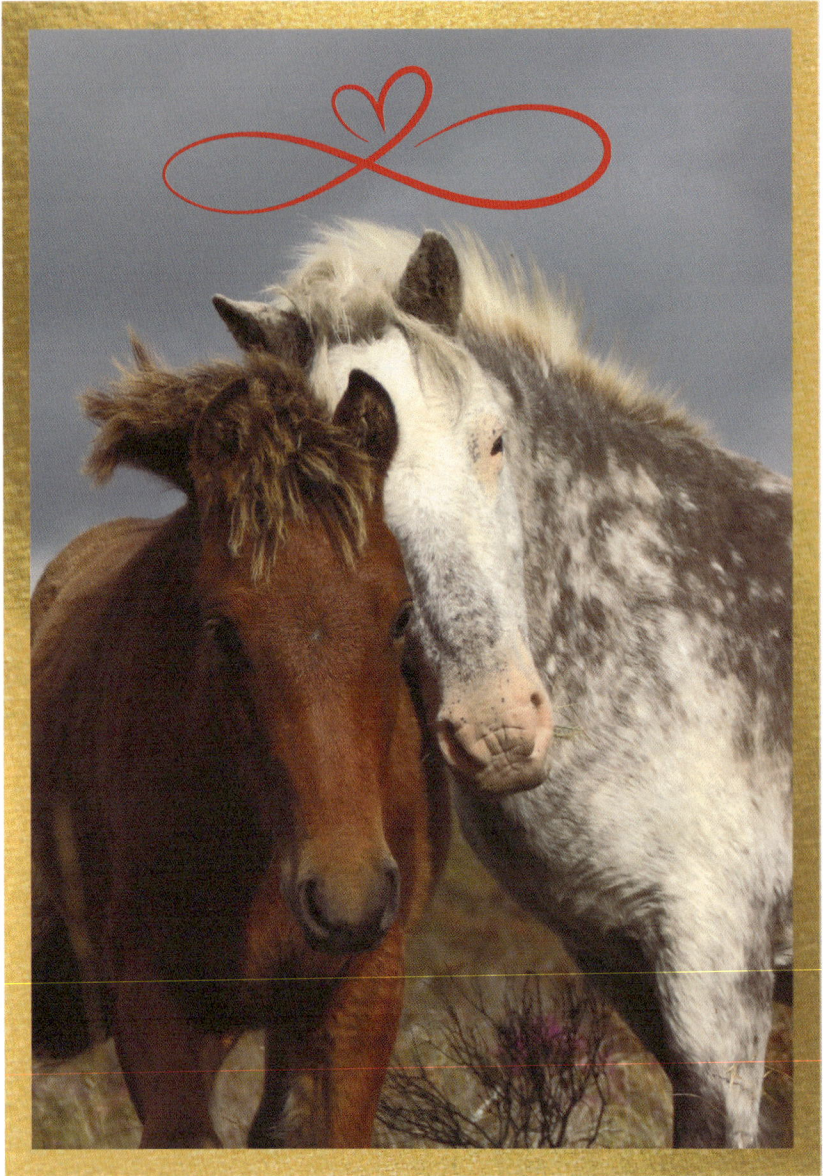

Let's never be apart!

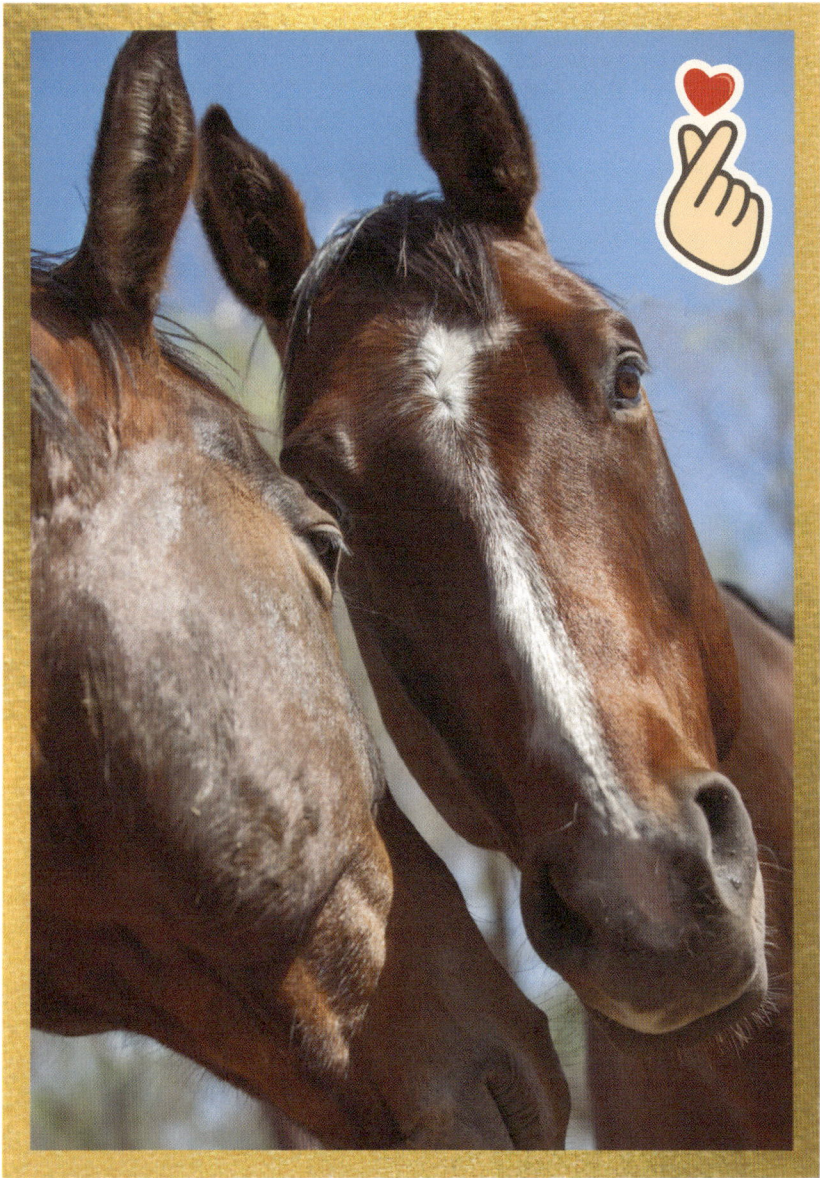

Hi my friend. Long time no see

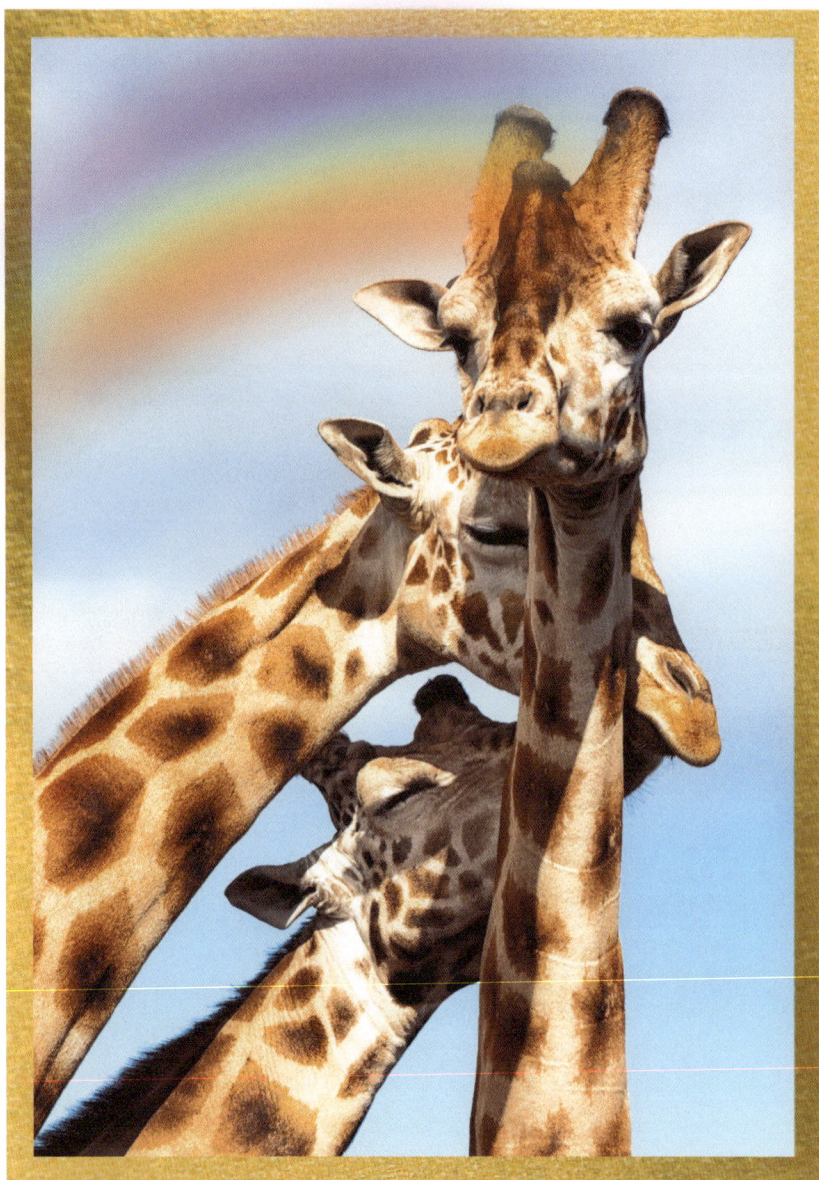

Love in a family

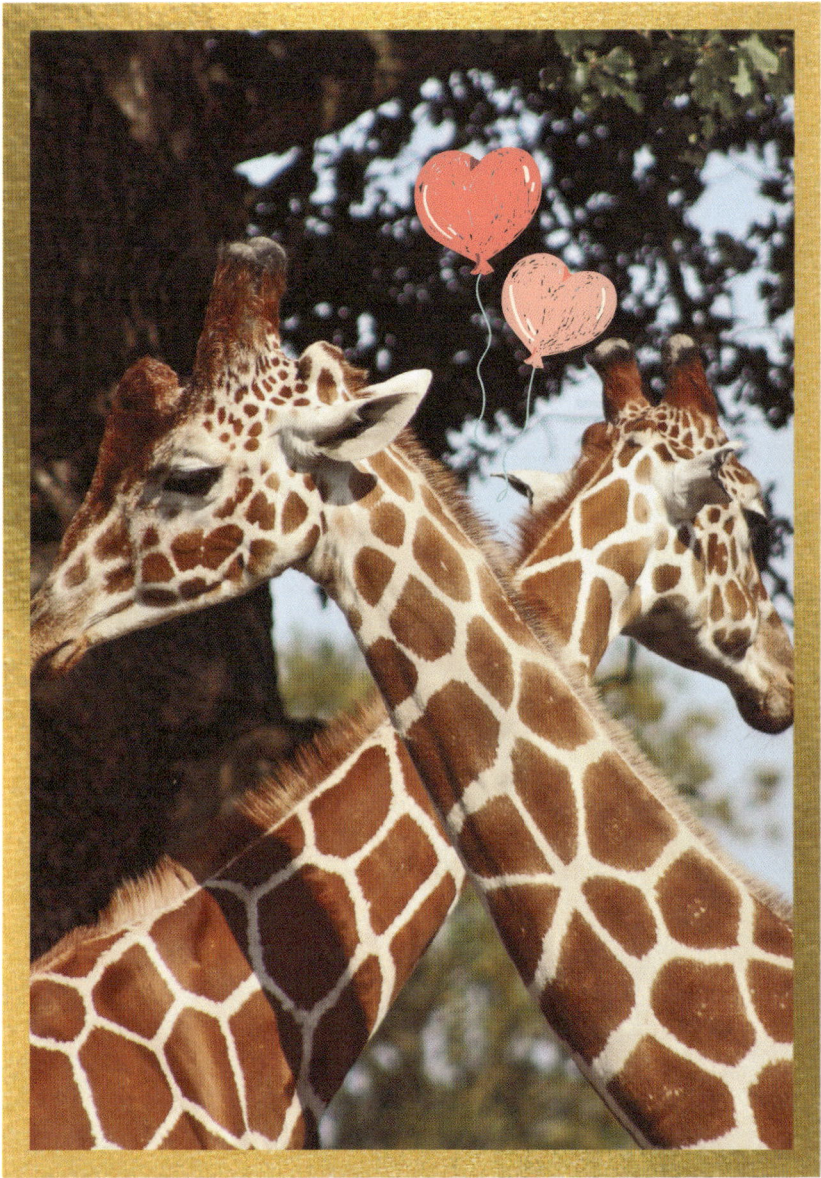

Do you love me?

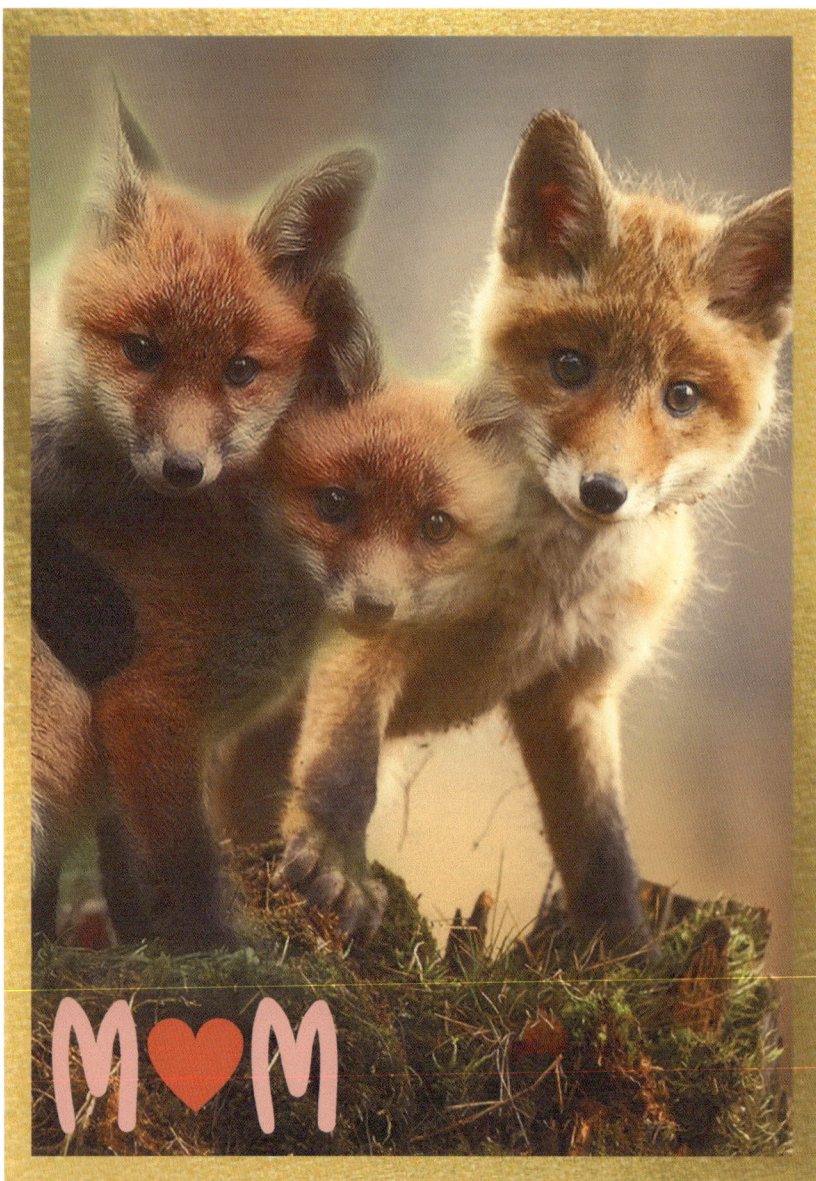

M♥M

We are waiting for mom

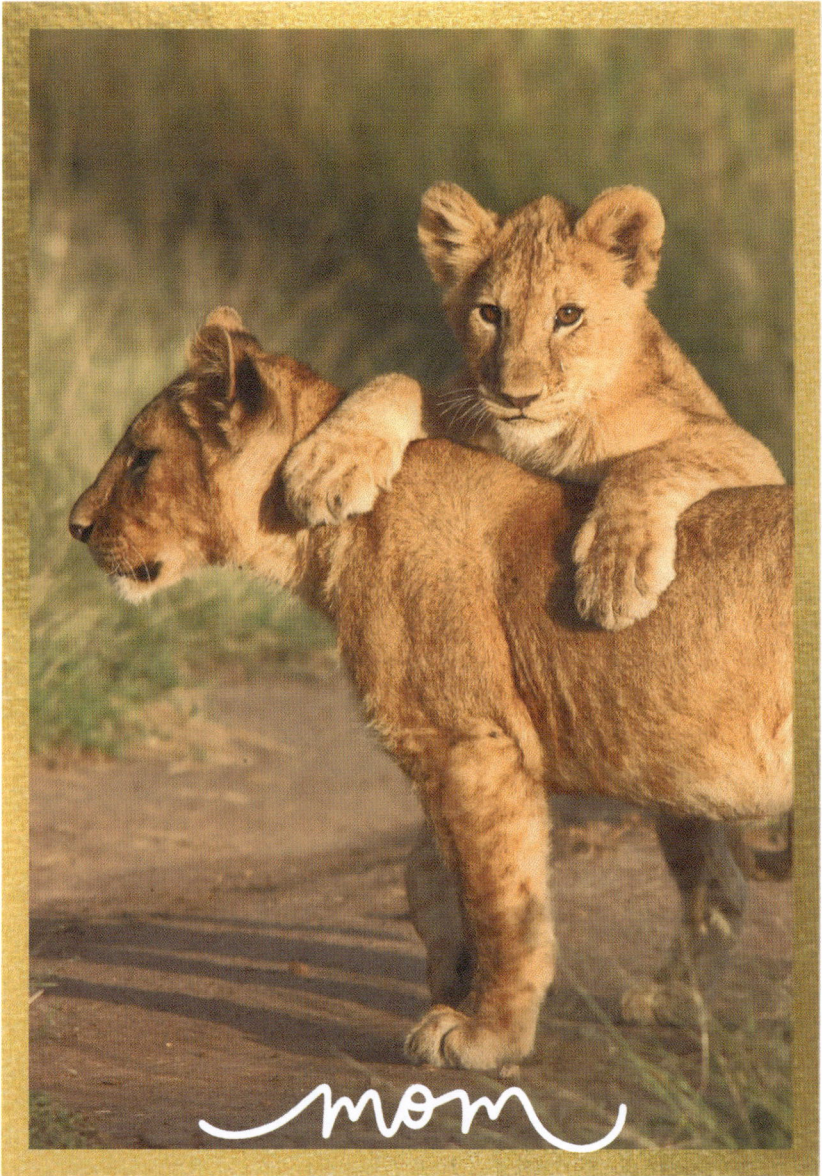

mom

Same here

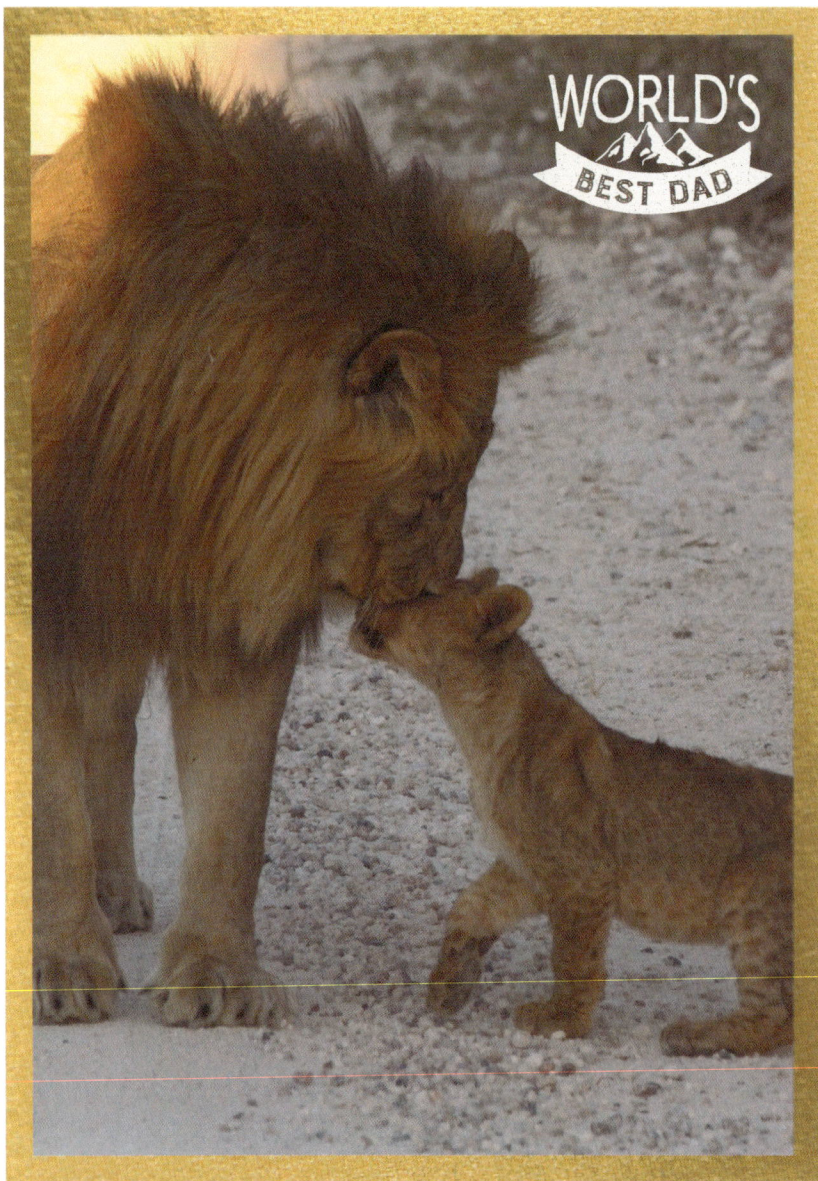

WORLD'S
BEST DAD

Dad loves you too

Dear Friend,

We hope you thoroughly enjoyed this cuddling animals picture book.

As a way of saying thank you for your support of our creation, we would love to send you a bonus gift which you will love!

You can either click on this link:

https://prodigious-thinker-229.ck.page/22314404e3

Or scan the QR code below to claim your free gift.

We would appreciate if you can leave us a review to encourage our work.

Yours Sincerely,
Dana Wee & Team

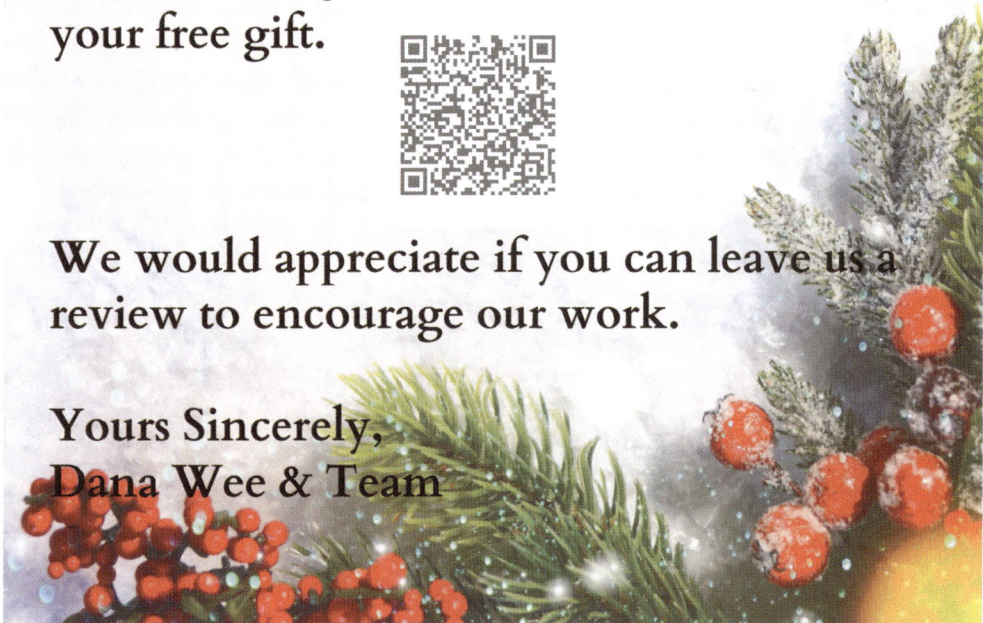

Printed in Dunstable, United Kingdom

66474101R00025